Mind Maps of Pharmacovigilance Basics

Amrita Akhouri

First Edition, 2015

Mind Maps of Pharmacovigilance Basics
Copyright © 2015 Amrita Akhouri

Contents

"Dedicated to my loving parents and most humbly to all my readers"

PREFACE

This book would be useful to anyone who wishes to enrich his/her knowledge on the fundamentals of pharmacovigilance. I ardently hope that this book would prove to be a true help to all those who are seeking to learn and grow in the field of pharmacovigilance.

Some of the readers might wonder what prompted me to write this book when there are several books already available on Pharmacovigilance basics.

In my opinion, there is a need for an organized study material which talks about the subject at the foundation level and presents the content in a form which is easy for the readers to understand/revise quickly. Hence, this book offers the readers a unique organized study material which comprises of mind maps, flow charts, short notes, text explanation and glossary thus, presenting the intricate concepts of the subject in a very simple manner. Over and above the core subject, this book also throws some light on careers in the field of pharmacovigilance which will be very helpful for the candidates preparing for job interviews in this field.

Any suggestion/feedback for improving the contents and making the book more user friendly is welcome. You can write to me at aakhouri6@gmail.com or amrita@crinov.com

One

INTRODUCTION TO DRUG DEVELOPMENT PROCESS

1.1 Learnings from the Chapter

- *Definition and concept of Drug and Disease*

- *Understanding of basis of treatment*

- *Drug development process overview in detail which includes drug discovery, pre-clinical study, clinical study and market study*

- *INDA and NDA details*

1.2 Introduction

Disease is anything which affects the proper functioning of the body and drugs are used to cure disease. **Fig: Introduction to Drug & Disease** depicts the improvement in the condition of the diseased person and restoration of the person's health after the drug was administered. Or, we can say that the equilibrium of the body (which was disturbed due to the diseased condition) got restored/established with the help of drug administration in the diseased body.

Drugs are usually distinguished from endogenous biochemicals as they are administered from external source in the body, for example, insulin is called a hormone when it is synthesized by the pancreas inside the body, but if it is introduced into the body from outside, it is called a drug.

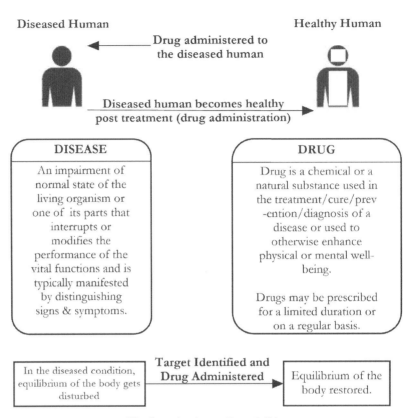

Fig: Introduction to Drug & Disease

1.3 Drug Development Process

Drug development process is basically bringing out a new medicinal product into the market. On an average, it takes about 10 - 15 years to develop a drug from its discovery to getting it approved for making it available in the market for its usage.

Drug development process can be divided into (Refer to **Fig - Drug Development process**):

- Discovery phase

- Pre-clinical phase

- Clinical phase

- Market phase

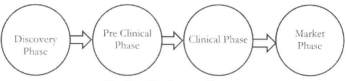

Fig: Drug Development Process

1.4   Drug Discovery phase

Discovery phase is the first phase of drug development process which includes the following (refer to **Fig - Discovery Phase Overview**):

- Target molecule selection (selection of the molecule responsible for disease)

- Lead discovery (Selection of potential/suitable compounds that might act against these target molecules)

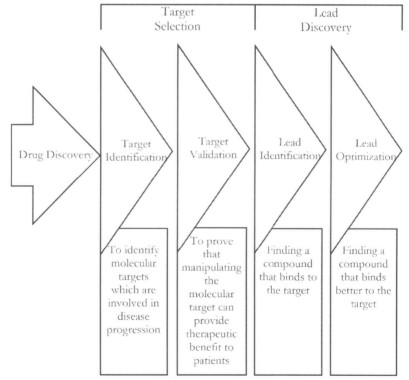

Fig: Discovery Phase Overview

Once a potential/suitable compound is identified it is modified in several ways to make it best suited compound to act against the target molecule. Tests are done in cellular and animal models to learn more about the compound's mechanisms of action against a particular target molecule. Once the research shows successful results, the compound moves into preclinical research.

Earlier, most of the drugs have been discovered either by identifying the active ingredient from traditional remedies or by serendipitous discovery, but now the scenario has changed as enough information is available about human genome and shapes of molecules at atomic level, so it is possible to control disease at the molecular and physiological level.

1.5   Basis of Treatment

Understanding the disease and the underlying cause of the disease is a pre-requisite for development of a drug/treatment. (Refer to the **Fig - Basis of Treatment**)

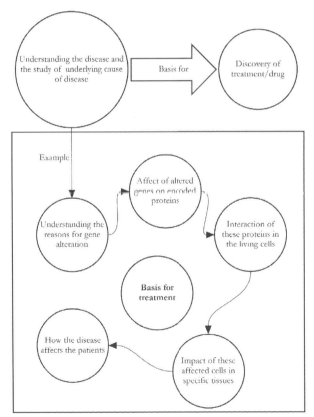

Fig: Basis of Treatment

1.6 Molecular basis of disease

Molecular basis of disease helps to understand the molecular mechanisms by which disease genes function, regardless of the type of disease. This can be done through variety of techniques like basic molecular, biochemical, cell biological techniques, proteomics and structural analyses.

1.7 Target identification

A drug target is the specific binding site of a drug in vivo through which the drug exerts its action. So, the disease mechanism is studied using cellular and genetic approaches, in order to identify potential drug targets. Various techniques used for target identification is described in **Fig- Techniques of target Identification**.

Techniques of Target Identification		
Genomics (Study of genome)	Proteomics (Study of proteome)	Bioinformatics (Science of collecting and analyzing biological data)
Knowledge of genome facilitates the identification of new biologial targets. Genomics evolution occurred through: a)Automation - results in a significant increase in the number of experiments that could be constructed in a given time. (eg. DNA sequencing) b) Informatics- the ability to transform raw data into meaningful information by applying computerized techniques for managing, analyzing, and interpreting data.	• The word "proteome" is a blend of "protein" and "genome". • The study of protein is required with the study of genes to understand the complexity of biological system. Therefore, the analysis of proteins (including protein-protein, protein-nucleic acid, and protein-ligand interactions) will be of utmost importance to target discovery.	•Systematically searching for paralogs (related proteins within an organism) of known drug targets helps in identifying new targets. (eg. possibility of modification of an existing drug to bind to the paralog). •Using gene expression microarrays and gene chip technologies, a single device can be used to evaluate and compare the expression of up to 20000 genes of healthy and diseased individuals at once.

Fig: Techniques of target identification

1.8   Target validation

demonstrates that a particular target is relevant to the disease being studied. Genes and their protein products that are highly expressed in disease tissues, but have low expression in normal tissues, become obvious potential targets for therapy. Validation can be done on cellular level, molecular level and whole animal model level for modulation of a desired target in disease patients (Refer to **Fig- target validation**).

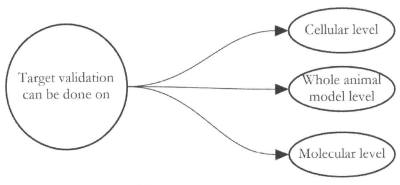

Fig: Target validation

1.9   Lead Discovery

Lead Discovery includes the following (depicted in the **Fig - Lead Discovery**):

  · Lead Identification (find a compound that binds to the target)

  · Lead Optimization (find a compound that binds better to the target)

Lead Discovery

Lead compound is a chemical that has phamacological/biological activity likely to be therapeutically useful, but may still have sub-optimal structure that requires modification to fit better to the target.

Lead Identification

Identification of a chemical that can interact with the target and has the potential to impact the disease studied.

Lead identification can be done through:

•HTS (High-throughput screening)
In this method, large libraries of chemicals are tested for their ability to modify the target. This process enables researchers to conduct millions of biochemical, genetic or pharmacological tests and rapidly identify those chemical compound that modulate a particular biomolecular pathway.

•Structure based drug design
Three dimensional structures of compounds from virtual or physically existing libraries are docked into binding sites of target proteins with known or predicted structure. Once hits have been identified via the screening approach, these are validated by re-testing them and checking the purity and structure of the compounds

Lead Optimization

Once a "lead" has been identified, the next stage is to find compounds that are similar to the lead compound that might bind even better (optimization).

To assess similarities, the following properties are analyzed:
-Absorption, distribution, metabolism, excretion, toxicity (ADMET).

Lead optimization can be obtained by physiological/stereo electric modification of lead.

Fig: Lead discovery

Once the molecule is finalized for development, it goes through pre-clinical and clinical phase to get a final approval for general use in public. Most substances fail to complete the course, as few as 1 in 10,000 undergo the entire program and reach the market.

1.10 Pre-Clinical Phase

In this phase, research in animal model, ex vivo experiments, in vivo experiments takes place to check the safety and efficacy of new potential compound which is carried out according to regulatory guidelines. Wide ranging dosages of the compounds are introduced to the cell line or animal in order to obtain preliminary efficacy and pharmacokinetic information about the new molecule (Refer to **Fig - Animal Studies**).

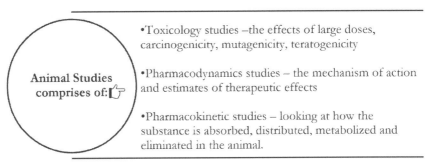

Fig: Animal studies

The results from preclinical research determine whether there is sufficient potential for a drug to proceed to testing in human clinical trials.

This ongoing program of pre-clinical studies synchronises with the clinical study programme. At each step in the clinical trial program, there must first have been reassuring information from animal studies. However, even at the time of application for a marketing authorization, there may be ongoing long-term animal studies (usually carcinogenicity studies).

1.11   Investigational New Drug Application (INDA)

Investigational New Drug Application (INDA)

Pre – clinical research tries to ensure that human will not be exposed to unreasonable risks in early phase clinical studies and this evidence is presented to health authority through IND (Investigational New Drug) application. Before starting experiments with new compound into humans, the company must file an Investigational New Drug (IND) application with the relevant authorities. Once the relevant health authorities have reviewed and approved a company's application, a process that usually takes at least one month, the drug may enter the first phase of human trials. All human research must then be approved by the ethics committee of the institution at which the study is conducted.

IND is submitted to Health authorities when the sponsor has completed satisfactory pre-clinical research to determine that it is safe to use the new molecule in human.

1.12   Clinical Phase

The clinical studies test the potential treatments (drug, device or biologics like vaccines) in human volunteers or patients to see whether they should be further investigated or approved for wider use in the general population. This is an integral part of drug development process and also required by regulatory authorities before a new treatment is brought into the market

The main objective of research is to demonstrate efficacy and acceptable safety in the intended population (Refer to **Fig - Phases of clinical studies and Fig - Clinical studies phases I-III**).

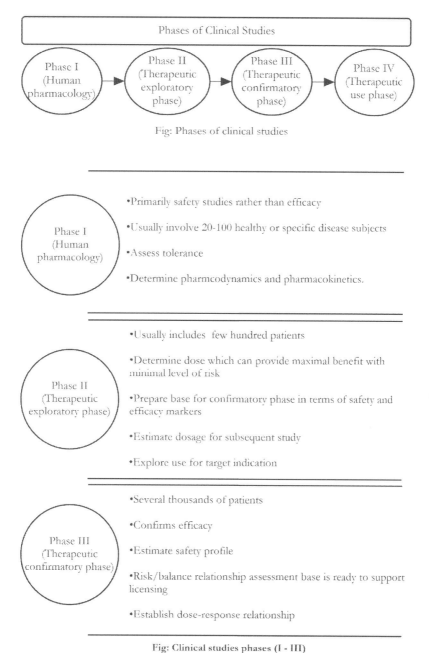

Fig: Phases of clinical studies

Phase I (Human pharmacology)
- Primarily safety studies rather than efficacy
- Usually involve 20-100 healthy or specific disease subjects
- Assess tolerance
- Determine pharmcodynamics and pharmacokinetics.

Phase II (Therapeutic exploratory phase)
- Usually includes few hundred patients
- Determine dose which can provide maximal benefit with minimal level of risk
- Prepare base for confirmatory phase in terms of safety and efficacy markers
- Estimate dosage for subsequent study
- Explore use for target indication

Phase III (Therapeutic confirmatory phase)
- Several thousands of patients
- Confirms efficacy
- Estimate safety profile
- Risk/balance relationship assessment base is ready to support licensing
- Establish dose-response relationship

Fig: Clinical studies phases (I - III)

1.13 New Drug Application (NDA)

New Drug Application (NDA)

Following the completion of Phase III clinical trials, company analyses and ensures that the data gathered during trial successfully demonstrates both safety and effectiveness. Then the company submits a registration dossier (NDA) with the authorities in each country where it wants permission to market the drug. The NDA contains all the scientific information that the company has gathered. The application submitted for marketing authorization is known as New Drug Application (NDA) in the US and Marketing Authorization Application for rest of the world (MAA in all countries except US). There is an active approval process for an NDA unlike IND. The clinical trials usually continue during the registration review period, and Phase IV studies are set up after marketing.

ANDA (Abbreviated New Drug Application) is used for generic drugs.

1.14 Market Phase (Phase IV - Therapeutic use phase)

Due to controlled clinical trials it is not possible to detect all effects related to the drug during trial and hence the post marketing safety system enables to detect serious, unexpected adverse reactions and to take required actions. Phase IV trials could be small open-label trials or massive scale multicentre double blind trials involving a comparator.

Market Phase
(Phase IV -
Therapeutic use
phase)

•Long term study which occurs after the Marketing authorization is granted for the new medicinal product and the new product is placed onto the market.

•Additional information for safety and efficacy profile

•Refined risk/benefit relationship understanding in general / special population and special environment

•Refined dosing recommendation

•Identifying rare ADR

• Marketing research or pharmaeconomic studies in relation to competitor drugs to assist sales

• Particular children's studies

• To investigate a specific Adverse Event or unexpected signal occurring during post-marketing

Fig: Clinical studies phase IV

Drug Development Process - Overview

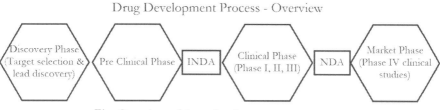

Fig: Overview of drug development process

Each step in the clinical research program is heavily regulated. Before introducing the new medicinal product in human, there is an assessment done by the regulatory authorities of all the animal and in vitro studies. Every clinical trial must be approved by the appropriate regulatory authorities and separately by ethics committees in each country based on summaries of the available evidence to date. All new relevant safety information arising from animal studies must be submitted to the authorities and the ethics committees during the clinical research program (and to the regulatory authorities if arising thereafter).

1.15   Safety review throughout drug development process

Throughout the clinical trials (pre & post registration), safety is paramount. Review of safety is performed by R&D and pharmacovigilance departments within the sponsor companies. However, CROs (Contract Research Organization) is often contracted out clinical trial activities by the sponsor companies but the responsibility for safety lies with the sponsor company. In addition, safety may be reviewed continuously by independent Drug Safety Monitoring Boards set up for specific studies. The importance of safety in clinical research is depicted in the **Fig: Safety in Drug Lifecycle**.

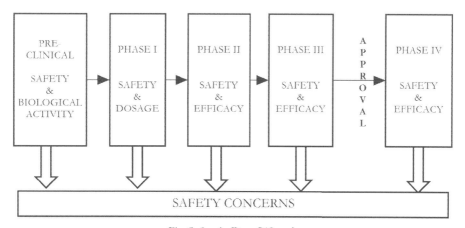

Fig: Safety in Drug Lifecycle

Two

HISTORY OF PHARMACOVIGILANCE

2.1   Learnings from the Chapter

Brief history/development of Pharmacovigilance

2.2   Introduction

The realization that it was important to have an independent evaluation of medicinal products before they are allowed on the market was reached at different times in different regions. However in many cases the realization was driven by tragedies, such as that with thalidomide in Europe in the 1960s.

Mentioned below is the brief history of development of Pharmacovigilance.

- 1959/61 - Thalidomide Disaster (Reports of fetal abnormalities) - 4000 -10000 cases

- 1962 - USA revised law requiring to prove safety and efficacy before issuing marketing authorization

- 1963 - British committee on safety of drug monitoring

- 1964 - UK started Yellow Card System (ADR reporting scheme) after the Thalidomide tragedy highlighted the need for routine monitoring of medicines.

- 1964-65 - National ADR reporting system UK, Australia, New Zealand, Canada, West Germany, Sweden.

- 1978 - WHO center moved from Geneva to Uppsala

- In India

  - 1986 - ADR monitoring system for India proposed (12 regional centers)

- 1997 - India joined WHO- ADR monitoring programme (3 centers AIIMS, KEM, JLN)

- 2004-2008 - National PV programme(2 zonal, 5 regional, 24 peripheral) overseen by CDSCO

- 2010 - Pharmacovigilance Programme of India (PVPI)

Three

PHARMACOVIGILANCE

3.1 Learnings from the Chapter

- *The concept of pharmacovigilance and needs of pharmacovigilance*

- *Methodologies of Pharmacovigilance*

- *Various aspects of Pharmacovigilance such as (products, factors, reports, tasks under PV, MSI, partners, etc).*

- *Few basic terms described (such as ADR, AE, SAE, Expected/Unexpected ADR).*

3.2 Introduction

With an intent to improve the public health, the field of Medicine is growing day by day in terms of new information, research, techniques, drugs etc, however, there are pros and cons which come as a result of such improvisations, for example, the medicines may lead to adverse reaction in the patients which may sometimes lead to death (refer to **Fig- Effects of Healthcare Products**). Hence, it is important to improve the patient's safety in terms of the use of medicines and this brings us to the topic of Pharmacovigilance.

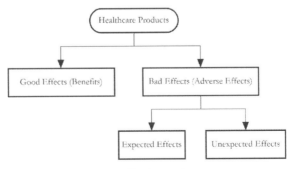

Fig: Effects of healthcare products

3.3 Pharmacovigilance

Pharmakon (Greek) = drug, Vigilare (Latin) = to keep watch.
According to WHO Definition: Pharmacovigilance (PV) is defined as the science and activities relating to the detection, assessment, understanding and prevention of adverse effects or any other drug-related problem.
Pharmacovigilance (PV) is also known as Drug Safety.

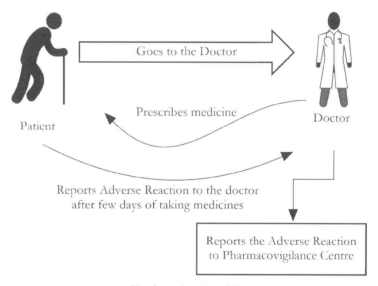

Fig: Introduction - PV

The figure (Introduction - PV) depicts the adverse reaction that may arise on administration of medicinal product to the patient who then reports the adverse reaction (effect) to the doctor and the doctor in turn reports the adverse reaction to the pharmacovigilance centre for further processing.

There are approved National and Regional Pharmacovigilance Centres which work on reported adverse effects (which are caused due to the use of medicinal products) to study the medicinal product activity and helps to take necessary actions related to medicinal product in terms of patient safety. The centre may be a hospital, an academic institution or as an independent facility such as a trust or foundation.

3.4 Need of Pharmacovigilance

Pharmacovigilance is needed to ensure safe, rational and ethical use of drugs/medicinal products (Refer to **Fig - Need of Pharmacovigilance**).

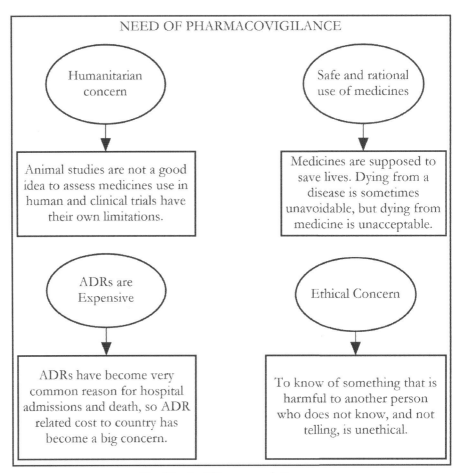

Fig: Need of Pharmacovigilance

3.5   Aim of Pharmacovigilance

· Improve patient care and safety

· Improve public health and safety

· Promote education and clinical training

· Early detection of unknown safety problems

· Detection of increase in frequency of (known) adverse reactions

· Identification of risk factors and possible mechanisms underlying adverse reactions

- Estimation of quantitative aspects of benefit/risk analysis and dissemination of information needed to improve drug prescribing and regulation

3.6 Tasks under Pharmacovigilance

- Timely data collection (pertaining to adverse events/adverse reaction), recording and notification

- Appropriate assessments (data completeness, seriousness, etc) of adverse events/adverse reaction

- Expedited and periodic reporting related to adverse event/adverse reaction

- Create appropriate structures for communication regarding the findings.

3.7 Scope of Pharmacovigilance

Although the controlled clinical trials are considered as a hallmark of demonstrating the efficacy of a drug, safety data available from those trials have well recognized limitations, for example; limited number of study subjects included in the trial, limited duration of drug exposure, etc. These limitations make it imperative for marketing authorization holder of a drug and regulatory authority to continue with collecting, analysing and interpreting data relevant to patient safety that becomes available after the drug is introduced into the market.

Hence, Pharmacovigilance applies throughout the life cycle of a medicinal product. It applies to the pre-approval stage as much as it applies to the post-approval stage (refer to **fig - PV in Pre/post authorization phases**)

Note: AE used for Adverse event and ADR used for Adverse Drug Reactions

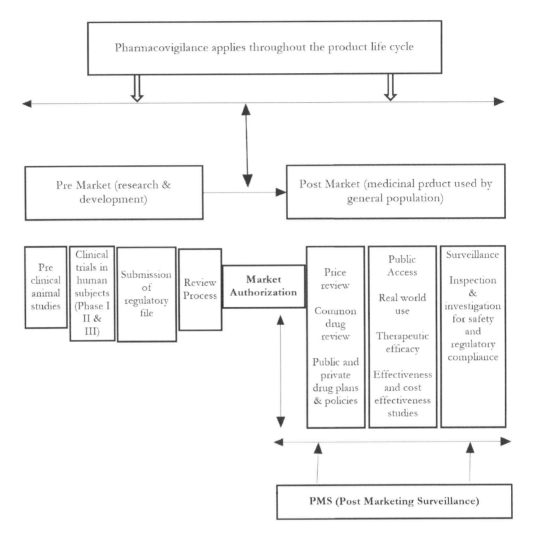

Fig: PV in Pre/Post authorization phases

3.8 Factors to be reported

These factors related to a medicinal product should be reported to the concerned manufacturer, regulatory authorities and other related bodies. (Refer to the **Fig - Factors to be reported**).

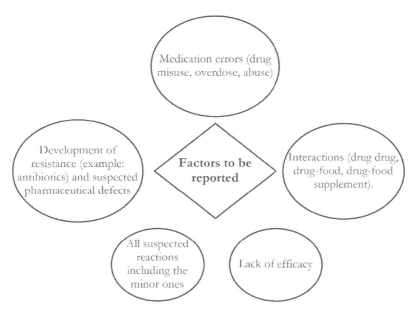

Fig: Factors to be reported

3.9   Products to be reported

These medicinal product should be reported to the concerned manufacturer, regulatory authorities and other related bodies in case of any adverse reaction/adverse event. (Refer to **Fig - Products to be reported**)

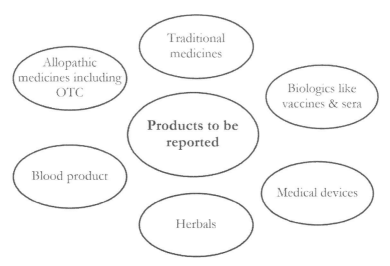

Fig: Products to be reported

3.10   MSI - Minimum Safety Information

According to WHO criteria, there is a set of basic information required before a case report becomes acceptable. The criteria is mentioned in the **Fig - MSI**.

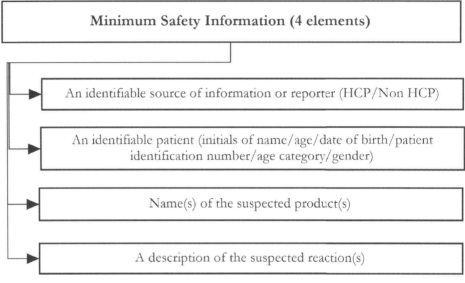

Fig: MSI

The four elements depicted in the **Fig - MSI** are called Minimum Safety Information (MSI) which makes any report valid for pharmacovigilance database. MSI helps in avoiding duplication of cases and detection of fraudulence and also helps in facilitating the follow up proccss.

If one or more of these four elements are missing, the case is not considered a valid AE report. Although there are no exceptions to this rule but there may be situation that may require a judgment call. For example, the term "identifiable" may not always be clear-cut. If a physician reports that he/she has a patient A taking drug X who experienced Z (an AE), but refuses to provide any specifics about patient A, the report is still a valid case even though the patient is not specifically identified. This is because the reporter has first-hand information about the patient and the patient is *identifiable* (i.e. a real person) to the physician.

Note: In different countries and regions of the world, drugs are sold under various trade names.

3.11 Medium Of Reporting

For reporting adverse effects, different types of forms are developed by the PV centres in the respective countries. To be effective, a reporting form needs to be in the local language and it should include information related to the concerned authority, for example: logo, address and contact details of issuing institution, etc. Apart from reporting forms, reporting can be done through telephone, fax, e-mail and internet. (Refer to **Fig: Medium of reporting**)

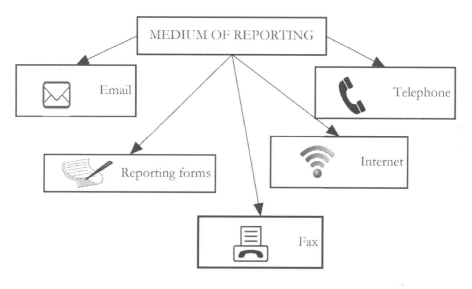

Fig: Medium of reporting

3.12 Where To Report

Adverse reaction/adverse event can be reported to manufacturers (MAH), regulatory authorities, PV centers and other bodies working under pharmacovigilance.

3.13 Methodology Of Pharmacovigilance

There are two methodologies of pharmacovigilance. They are referred to as Passive and Active methodologies (depicted in the **Fig: Pharmacovigilance Methodologies**)

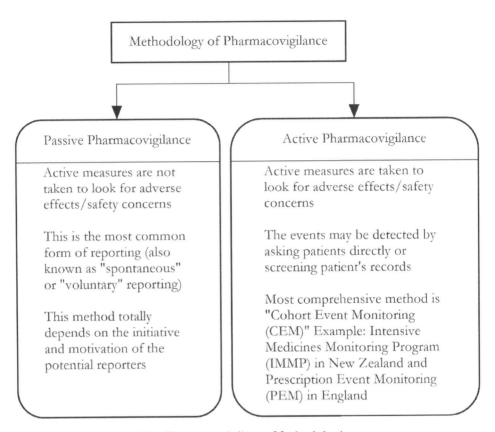

Fig: Pharmacovigilance Methodologies

3.14 Pharmacovigilance Process Overview (Generalized)

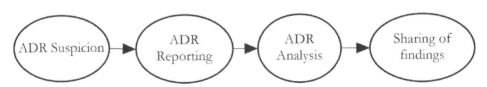

Fig: PV Process summarized

Case processing is a processing of ADR reports that the company receives from various sources.

- Once the case of adverse event/reaction is received from any source (Telephone, fax, email, licensing agreement, form, the regulators or other companies), the case is checked for 4 valid criteria i.e. minimum safety information.

- If the case is valid, the adverse event/reaction coding is done using standardized terminology from MedDRA and then the case is evaluated for its seriousness criteria by triage team.

- A unique identity number is assigned to each individual case.

- Then the case is sent to the safety associate for data entry. The work of case processing team starts now.

- The safety associate enters the case into safety database, performs coding (for disease and medicines) and writing narratives of the case.

- In case of any query he/she seeks the follow up information from the reporter.

- After the data entry, the case is assigned to the QC (quality control) team, where the QC person checks the work done by Safety associates.

- The case moves in the workflow to the Medical Reviewer who assesses the case for Medical aspects, performs the causality assessment (relationship of given ADR and specific drug) and gives a company comment on each case.

- Next step is Signal detection (identifying signals i.e. potential indicator of new ADR) and risk management plan (risk assessment and risk minimization plan) post which the analysis is completed through various methods like statistical methods (e.g. t-test for the comparison of mean), data manipulation (e.g. tabular and graphics).

- Now the case is ready for submission to the regulatory authority and communication to other partners. The submission team submits the Case to the regulatory authority according to the local requirement.

The case processing steps are depicted in **Fig - PV overview**.

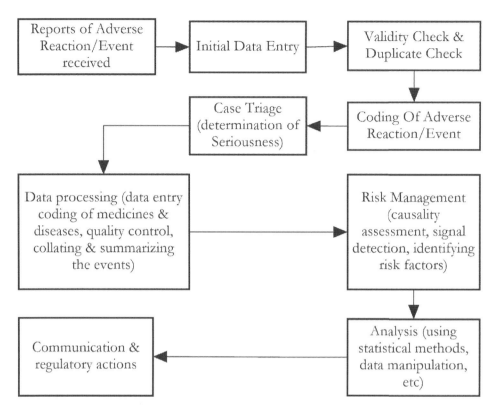

Fig: PV overview (generalized)

3.15 Partners In Pharmacovigilance

There are a wide range of partners under the PV system and each one of them have a role in the system. (Refer to **Fig - Partners in Pharmacovigilance**)

Some important terms used in PV which we must understand very clearly to make a strong foundation in pharmacovigilance.

3.16 Adverse Drug Reaction (ADR)

Any substance that has a potential to produce therapeutic benefits can be associated to some unwanted effects (mild to severe). For example a person has taken a medicine for headache and he starts feeling uneasiness and excessive sweating after having medicine.

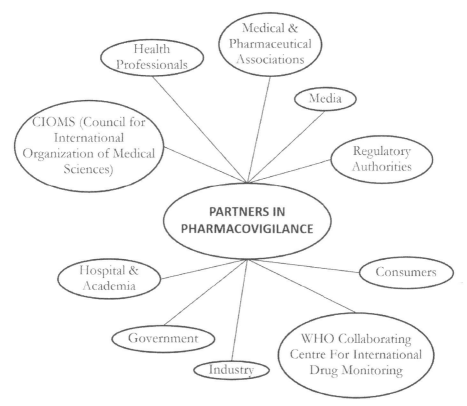

Fig: Partners in Pharmacovigilance

Regarding pre-approval product in clinical experience: all noxious and unintended responses to a medicinal product related to any dose should be considered adverse drug reactions.

The phrase "responses to a medicinal product" means that a causal relationship between a medicinal product and an adverse event is at least a reasonable possibility, i.e., the relationship cannot be ruled out.

Regarding marketed medicinal products, according to WHO definition:

A response to a drug which is noxious and unintended and which occurs at doses normally used in man for prophylaxis, diagnosis, or therapy of disease or for modification of physiological function.

Classifications of ADRs

ADR is very important as safe use of the medicinal product is a critical issue for pharmaceutical industry, doctors, pharmacist, regulatory authorities and public. ADR may occur immediately or after prolonged use after termination. Classification of ADR is depicted in **Fig - Classifications of ADRs**.

CLASSIFICATION OF ADRs	
Type A (Augmented) Reactions	**Type B (Bizarre) Reactions**
Dose related Extension of pharmacological effect Also called predictable or anticipated events Most frequent & less serious Example: Respiratory depression with opioids	Non dose related Also called pharmacologically unexpected, unpredictable or Idiosyncratic Adverse Reactions Generally more serious & less frequent Example: Skin rashes with antibiotics
Type C (Continuing) Reactions	**Type D (Delayed) Reactions**
Dose & time related Associated with long term use Example: NSAIDS (Nonsteroidal anti-inflammatory drugs) Induced Renal Failure	Apparent only sometime after use of drug Timing of these may make them more difficult to detect Example: Thalidomide in first trimester caused phocomelia limb defects
Type E (End of Use) Reactions	**Type F (Failure of Therapy) Reactions**
Associated with the withdrawal of a medicine Example: Insomnia, anxiety & perceptual disturbances following the withdrawal of benzodizepines	Failure of therapy which can be due to diverse causes such as inadequate information on the consumption, quality of drugs etc. Example: Antitubercular therapy

Fig: Classification of ADRs

Prevention of ADR

By taking the following steps, chances of ADR can be minimized/prevented.

- Avoid inappropriate drugs in the context of clinical conditions
- Use right dose, route ,frequency based on patient variables
- Elicit medication history and history of allergy
- Rule out drug interactions
- Adopt right technique of medication and follow adequate monitoring

3.17   Adverse Event (AE)

Any untoward medical occurrence experienced by a patient (or subject) that is administered with a medicinal product does not necessarily having causal relationship with the treatment.

So, in order to qualify as an AE, it is not necessary that a healthcare provider makes any determination about the causal link between the medical event and the drug exposure. An adverse event (AE) can therefore be any unfavourable and unintended sign (including an abnormal laboratory finding, for example), symptom, or disease temporally associated with the use of a medicinal product, whether or not considered related to the medicinal product.

ADR is subset of AE

All Adverse Drug Reactions are adverse events but all Adverse Events are not Adverse Drug Reactions.

The **principal difference** between an adverse event (AE) and an adverse drug reaction (ADR) is that a causal relationship is suspected for the latter, but is not required for the former. In this framework, adverse drug reactions are a subset of adverse event. (Refer to **Fig- ADR is subset of Adverse Event**).

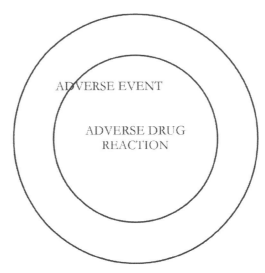

ADR - A Causal Role is Suspected
AE - Does not imply Causality

Fig: ADR is the subset of Adverse Event

Dimensions of AE

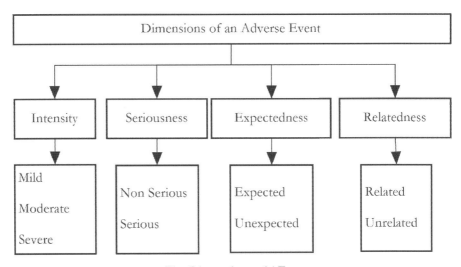

Fig: Dimensions of AE

The term "severe" is often used to describe the intensity (severity) of a specific event (as in mild, moderate, or severe myocardial infarction). The event itself, may be of relatively minor medical significance (such as severe headache) while the term "serious," is based on patient's event outcome or action criteria. Seriousness (not severity) serves as a guide for defining regulatory reporting obligations.

Serious	Severe
Defined as a regulatory definition	Defined as an intensity classification (mild, moderate, severe)

3.18   Serious Adverse Event (SAE)

Definition and Criteria of SAE

An adverse event is considered serious if it meets one or more of the following criteria.

- Death

- Life threatening Situation (Life-threatening in the definition of a serious adverse event or serious adverse reaction refers to an event in which the patient/subject was at risk of death at the time of the event. It does not refer to an event which hypothetically might have caused death if it were more severe.)

- Requires inpatient hospitalization or prolongation of existing hospitalization

- Disability (the condition of being unable to do things in the normal way)

- Congenital anomalies / Birth defect (structural or functional anomalies, including metabolic disorders, which are present at the time of birth.)

- Important medical event (refers to which does not fit into other outcomes but require treatment to prevent one or the other outcomes. Example- allergic bronchospasm (serious breathing problem) requires treatment in emergency room.

Outcomes of SAE

Outcomes of SAE (worst to most favourable outcome)

1. Death
2. Recovered with sequel (leading to some other event)
3. Not Recovered
4. Unknown (may be recovering or may not be recovering)
5. Recovering
6. Recovered

Fig: Outcomes of SAE

Note: Surgical procedures are not AEs/SAEs as per se, the condition for which surgical procedures are performed may be an AEs/SAEs which has to be reported. Surgical procedures are therapeutic measures of a condition requiring surgery. Surgical procedures planned prior to randomization and conditions leading to these measures are not AEs (medical history).

3.19 Expected ADR

An ADR whose nature, severity, specificity, or outcome is consistent with the applicable product information (e.g., Investigator's Brochure for an unapproved investigational medicinal product/package insert or product monograph for marketed product).

3.20 Unexpected ADR

An ADR whose nature, severity, specificity, or outcome is not consistent with the applicable product information (e.g., Investigator's Brochure for an unapproved investigational medicinal product/package insert or product monograph for marketed product).

When a Marketing Authorization Holder (MAH) is uncertain whether an ADR is expected or unexpected, the ADR should be treated as unexpected. An expected ADR with a fatal outcome should be considered unexpected unless the local/regional product labeling specifically states that the ADR might be associated with a fatal outcome.

3.21 Basic flowchart of processing of AEs/ADRs (During clinical trial and post marketing space)

Clinical Trial

In the clinical trial process, when a subject experiences any adverse event/reaction, he informs to his investigator at clinical trial site, investigator reports this adverse event/reaction information to CRO and CRO reports the same to the PV department of pharmaceutical company (sponsor) for processing of adverse event/reaction and further company reports the adverse event/reaction information to the regulatory authority. In some cases investigator reports directly to Pharmaceutical company (in case no CRO in middle). Refer to **Fig - Generalized process flow of Adverse Event/reaction -during clinical trials.**

Post marketing space

In case of post marketing space, patient informs adverse reaction to health care professionals (HCP) such as physician/pharmacist/nurses/dentist/coroner (an official who holds inquest into violent, sudden and suspicious death), then health care professional reports the ADR

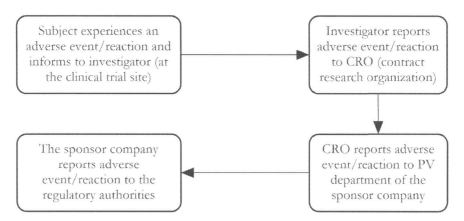

Fig: Generalized process flow of Adverse Event/Reaction - during clinical trials

to affiliates of pharmaceutical company and the affiliates inform the same to PV department of pharmaceutical company for further processing of ADR and reporting to Regulatory authorities. (Refer to **Fig - Generalized Process Flow of Adverse Event/reaction - During Post Marketing Space**)

Affiliates are officially attached bodies to the pharmaceutical companies which are present all across the world. Affiliates plays as a link between local regulatory body and PV department as they know local regulatory regulations (regulatory regulations varies from country to country) and thus helps PV department in processing of adverse reactions efficiently. Informing the affiliates about ADR is considered as informing to the pharmaceutical company.

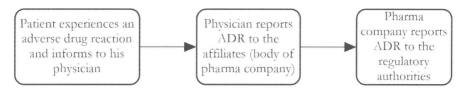

Fig: Generalized process flow of Adverse Event/Reaction - during post marketing space

Four

REPORTING OF ADVERSE REACTIONS AND ADVERSE EVENTS

4.1   Learnings from the chapter

- *Importance of reporting adverse effects.*

- *Different types of reporters, reports, sources of reports and reporting forms.*

- *Reporting timeframes during clinical trials and post marketing space.*

- *Concept of SUSARs*

4.2   Introduction

The continuous surveillance of adverse events/reaction, once the medicinal product has been marketed and given to many more patients (in comparison to controlled clinical trial subjects), is the only way to reveal a complete pattern of adverse effects related to the medicinal product; for example, some cases of rare adverse effects may be serious enough to warrant additional precautions or even withdrawal of a medicinal product from the market.

4.3   Importance of Reporting

Two scenarios are being discussed here to develop a clear understanding of the importance of reporting. First: the impact of not reporting and second: the impact of reporting.

Impact of not reporting

Drug prescribed to a patient leads to an adverse effect in patient which if not reported can have various consequences as depicted in the **Fig - Impact of not reporting**.

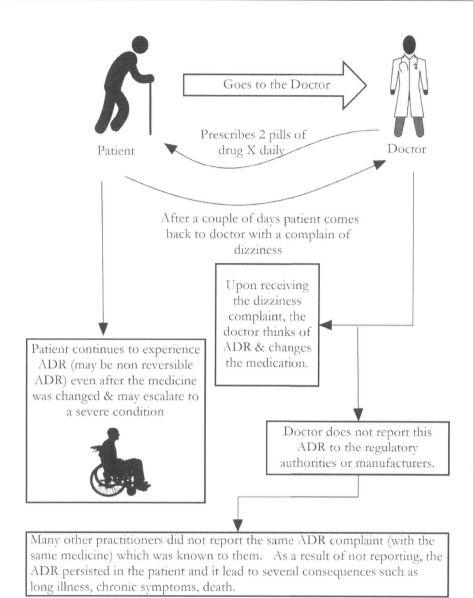

Fig: Scenario - Impact of Not Reporting

Impact of reporting

Drug prescribed to a patient leads to an adverse effect in patient which if reported, can be of helpful consequence as depicted in the **Fig- Impact of reporting**

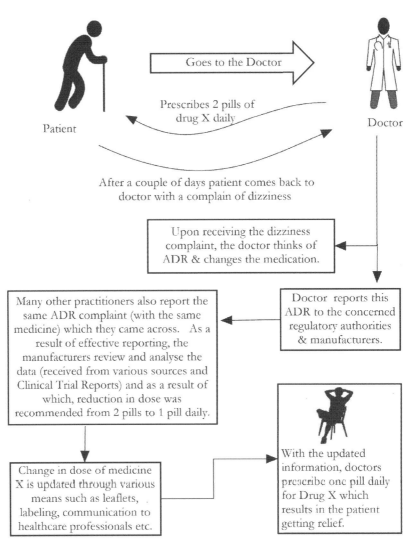

Fig: Scenario - Impact of Reporting

4.4   Effective Reporting

Effective reporting of adverse effects helps the PV system in monitoring activities of a marketed medicinal product by adding information about the medicinal product (Refer to **Fig - Benefits of Effective Reporting**). It is compulsory for pharmaceutical manufacturers to ensure that the suspected adverse reactions related to their products are reported to the competent authority as they are primarily responsible for their product safety

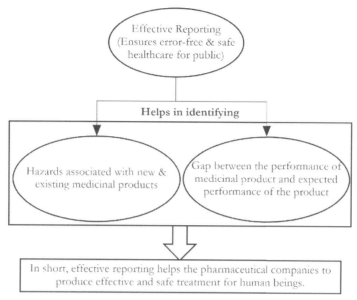

Fig: Benefits of Effective Reporting

4.5 Who all can report?

Basically anyone can report the adverse reaction related to a medicinal product. Some of those are depicted in the **Fig: Who all can report**.

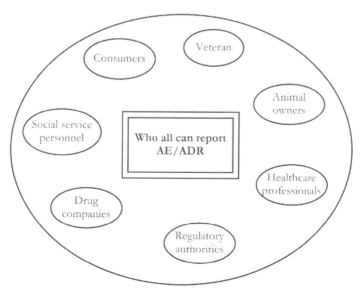

Fig: Who all can report

4.6 Sources Of Adverse Event/Reactions Reports

There are various sources from where the ADR and AE reports can be obtained. These sources can be classified as unsolicited and solicited source. (Refer to **Fig -Sources of ADR/AE reports**)

4.7 Unsolicited source

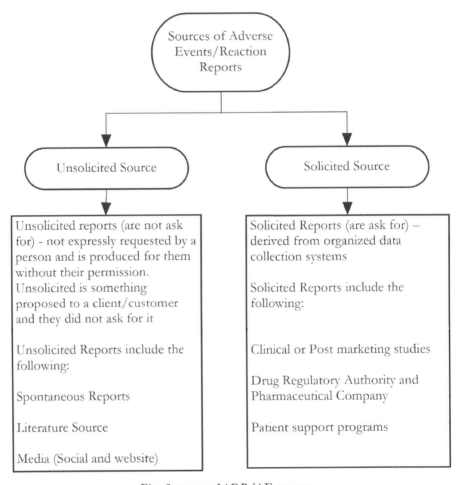

Fig: Sources of ADR/AE reports

Spontaneous Reports

An unsolicited communication by a healthcare professional or a non-healthcare professional to a competent authority, marketing authorization holder or other organization(e.g. regional Pharmacovigilance Centre) that describes one or more suspected adverse reactions in a patient who was given one or more medicinal products and that does not derive from a study or any organized data collection systems.

Adverse reaction reports received from the consumers should be considered spontaneous reports irrespective of any subsequent medical confirmation. These reports will be evaluated for medical aspects so that expedited reporting to regulatory authority can be decided. Even if reports do not fulfill regulatory requirement, report should be retained.

Healthcare professionals are the preferred source of information in pharmacovigilance, for instance physician, pharmacists, dentists, nurses and other health workers may also administer or prescribe drugs and they should report the relevant experiences.

Literature Source

The pharmaceutical company does a literature screening process (weekly) to identify adverse reactions related to medicinal products which are published in the medical and scientific literature and these adverse reactions must be reported by the company in a similar way to the regulatory authorities.

Literature reports have more scientific weightage in comparison to spontaneous reports. Many doctors report series of cases that they have come across, instead of individual case report. Normally, literature reports contain detailed and medically confirmed information. Hence, it is much more important for signal detection process and it is also one of the mandatory requirement for regulatory submission of periodic reports.

Media

If MAH comes across any adverse reaction regarding their medicinal product on a social media or other websites (which MAH does not manage), MAH should analyze the case and should check if it is reportable to concerned authority or not.

MAH should provide facility on their website for ADR data collection regarding their product. For example, providing reporting forms to report ADR, providing appropriate contact details for direct communication. Cases from internet should be considered spontaneous reports.

4.8   Solicited Sources

Clinical/post - marketing studies

Clinical study (or trial) refers to an organized program to determine the safety and/or efficacy of a drug (or drugs) in patients. The design of a clinical trial will depend on the drug and the phase of its development. It is an interventional study and various adverse reaction/event reports may arise during these studies which are reportable. In contrast post marketing studies are combination of interventional (Phase IV) and non-interventional (observational) studies.

Pharmaceutical Company and Drug Regulatory Authority

The marketing of many medicines increasingly takes place through contractual agreements between two or more companies, which may market same product in the same or different countries/regions. Arrangements vary considerably with respect to inter-company communication and regulatory responsibilities. Overall, this can be a complex issue. In such relationships, it is very important that explicit licensing/contractual agreements specify the processes for exchange of safety information, including timelines and regulatory reporting responsibilities. Safety personnel should be involved in development of any agreements from the beginning. Processes should be in place to avoid duplicate reporting to the regulatory authority, e.g. assigning responsibility to one company for literature screening. Whatever the nature of the arrangement, the MAH is ultimately responsible for regulatory reporting. Therefore, every reasonable effort should be made between the contracting partners to minimize the data exchange period so as to promote compliance with MAH responsibilities.

The authorities in turn are required to report to each company anonymized information on the serious adverse reactions that they have received in relation to that company's marketed products. There are also requirements for companies to report spontaneous cases of serious adverse reactions that they have received from certain regulatory authorities to their own authorities. There are mechanisms in place to identify and remove duplicate reports.

Wherever there is a contractual agreement between two or more parties (companies) to share the drug safety information regarding a specific medicinal product, the companies are obliged to share the information. Refer to the **Fig: Contractual agreement between company A and B.**

Wherever there is no contractual agreement between two or more parties (companies), they are not obliged to share the drug safety information regarding a specific medicinal product. Refer to the **Fig: No contractual agreement between company A and B.**

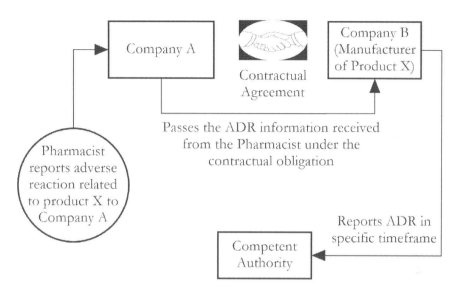

Fig: Contractual Agreement between Company A and B regarding
exchange of drug safety information related to product X

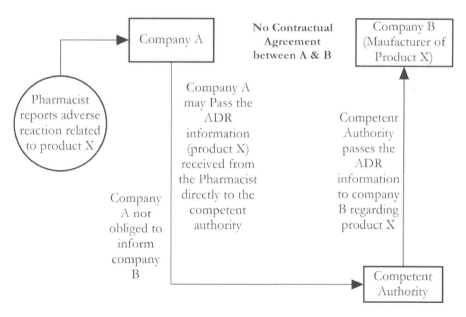

Fig: No Contractual Agreement between Company A and B regarding
exchange of drug safety information related to product X

Patient support programme

A patient support programme is an organised system where a MAH receives and collects information relating to the use of its medicinal products. Examples are post authorisation Patient support and disease management programmes, surveys of patients and healthcare providers, information gathering on patient compliance, or compensation/re-imbursement schemes.

4.9   Types of Reporting Forms

To report ADRs, various reporting forms are available for general population and marketing authorization holders. They are voluntary forms and mandatory forms described in **Fig-Reporting Forms**.

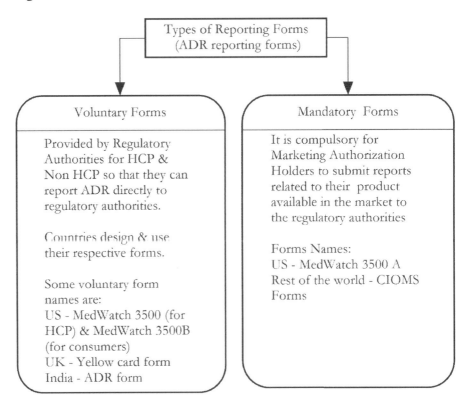

Fig: Reporting Forms

4.10   Modes of Reporting

Reporting can be done manually or electronically (Refer to **Fig - Modes of Reporting**). E2B (electronic reporting of adverse event) is the standard which, ensures that the information on suspected ADR is easily transferred and therefore it facilitates uniformity and high quality with regard to the content and format of ICSR (Individual Case Safety Report). E2B uses XML application for transition.

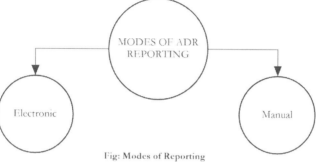

Fig: Modes of Reporting

4.11   What to Report

Reporting of adverse event/reaction during clinical trial and post marketing depends on various factors like seriousness, expectedness and causality. The following **fig - What to Report** depicts the same.

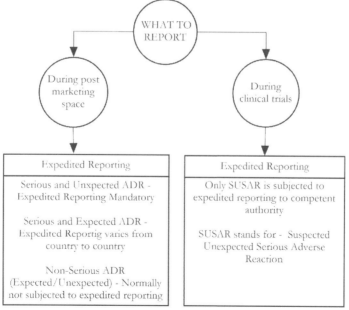

Fig: What to Report

Expedite means 'faster', the ADR'S which are unexpected, serious, fatal, & life threatening should be reported faster as possible. So these are subjected to expedited reporting. So, an expedited report would be a "Report" meeting the criteria for rapid transmission to a Competent Authority.

The purpose of expedited reporting is to make regulators, investigators, and other appropriate people aware of new, important information on serious reactions.

During Post marketing space

An ADR is the one which occurs at the normal doses when used for diagnosis, treatment, precaution or to explore the physiological functions & is always related to drug. So in case of PMS study all the adverse effects have to be reported as ADR.
Note:

- *Reporting requirement related to the new drug - reporting of all suspected reactions (known or unknown, serious or not serious) including the minor ones.*

- *Under new EU Pharmacovigilance legislation, the reporting of non-serious adverse reactions (arose from EU countries) should be done within 90 days.*

- *All SAE and non SAE will be recorded in the safety database.*

During clinical trials

During clinical trial the causality assessment given by the investigator should not be downgraded by the sponsor. If the sponsor disagrees with the investigator's causality assessment, both the opinion of the investigator and the sponsor should be provided with the report. The expectedness of an adverse event/reaction shall be determined by the sponsor according to the reference document (refer to **Fig - Assessment of Adverse event/reaction in terms of seriousness, causality and expectedness during clinical trial**). The reference document includes investigator's brochure for a non-authorized investigational medicinal product and summary of product characteristics (SmPC) for an authorized medicinal product.

During clinical research with a medicinal product, there may be a causal link between the adverse reaction occurs with subject and the medicinal product administered to subject; this is known as SUSAR (**SUSAR** stands for **Suspected Unexpected Serious Adverse Reaction**) if the adverse reaction is both unexpected (not consistent with the applicable product information) and also meets the definition of a Serious Adverse Event/Reaction.
SUSAR must fulfill the following three criteria:

- The event must be **serious**

- There is an **adverse reaction**

- The adverse reaction must be **unexpected** (the nature and severity of the adverse reaction are **not in agreement with the product information as recorded in)**.

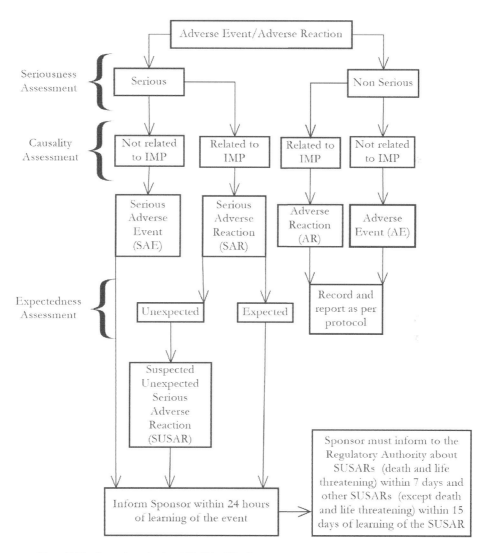

Note: IMP refers to Investigational Medicinal Product

Fig: Assessment of Adverse Event/Adverse Reaction in terms of seriousness, causality and expectedness during clinical trial

4.12 Documents assessing Expectedness/Unexpectedness and Listedness/Unlistedness

---

Documents assessing Expectedness/Unexpectedness and Listedness/Unlistedness

For an authorized medicinal product (post-marketing space):

- Global document –
- CCDS (Company Core Data Sheet) /CCSI (Company Core Safety Information)

- CCDS - A document prepared by the Marketing Authorization Holder containing, in addition to safety information, material relating to indications, dosing, pharmacology and other information concerning the product.

- CCSI is the reference information(present in CCDS) by which listed and unlisted are determined for the purpose of periodic reporting for marketed products, but not by which expected   and unexpected are determined for expedited reporting.

- Local document - document related to particular nation

USPI (US Package Insert), **SmPC** (Summary of Product Characteristics).

It may happen that molecule A is having 10 SmPCs but as a rule each molecule is always has one CCSI. Also, CCSI may contain the less safety information which is available in each and every SmPC but vice-a-verse is not true. So rarely it may happen the event is unlisted but may be expected as per the local label (SmPC). The purpose of expectedness/ labeledness is to assess the reportability of the case to health authorities, whereas listedness, based on CCSI is for the generation of periodic reports.

SO, in short,

Listedness is based on the global document i.e. CCSI which is the core information on safety profile of molecule available with MAH.

Expectedness is based on Local documents i.e. SmPC or PI which is a local label and is related to particular nation.

For an unauthorized medicinal product: the Investigator's Brochure

Investigator's Brochure can be defined as: A compilation of the clinical and non-clinical data known to date on the investigational product(s) that is relevant to the study of the investigational product (s) in human subjects.

4.13 Reporting Timeframe

MAH is obliged to report about the adverse reaction/events to the regulatory authorities in a specific timeframe. In case MAH is not compliant to this requirement, they would be facing some regulatory issues.

Reporting of SUSAR during clinical trials

In a clinical trial, SUSARs that are life-threatening or have fatal consequences must be reported to Regulatory authority and IRB/IEC at the latest, within 7 calendar days after the sponsor has become aware of them. All relevant information on the aftermath of this must be reported within a time period of a further 8 days. Other reports of SUSARs must be made within 15 calendar days (India- 14 calendar days) after the sponsor has become aware of them.

But the investigator at the clinical trial site has to inform all SAE immediately (within 24 hrs) to the sponsor (except those that the protocol and other relevant documents identify as not needing immediate reporting) and to Ethics Committee within 7 working days (Refer to **Fig - Reporting timeframe during clinical trial**).

Post marketing reporting

Reporter can report directly to the company marketing the product or to the regulatory authority but MAH has to report all Serious ADR (under legal obligation) to health authority within 15 calendar days (Refer to **Fig -Reporting timeframe during post marketing space**).

The Regulatory reporting time clock is considered to start on the date when any personnel of MAH first receive a case report that fulfills the minimum criteria as well as criteria of expedited reporting. This date should be considered as "Day 0".

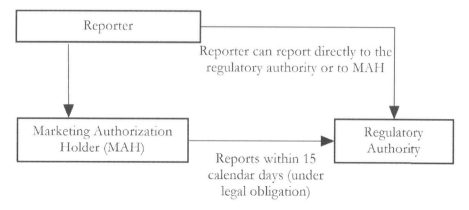

Fig: Reporting timeframe during post marketing space

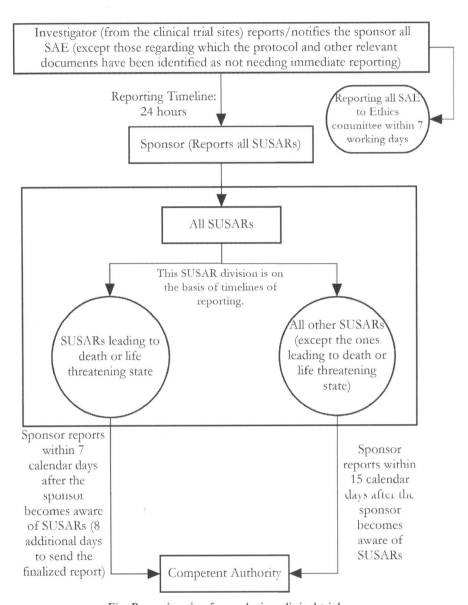

Fig: Reporting timeframe during clinical trial

4.14   Day Zero

Day zero is the date on which any personnel of an organization (MAH) or third party which has a contractual agreement with that organization, receives the case report/adverse reaction report (for the first time) that fulfills the minimum criteria as well as the criteria of expedited reporting.

Example: A patient reports an adverse reaction with only 3 MSI out of 4 MSI elements to a manufacturer on 5th October 2014 and gives 4th element of MSI on 7th October 2014. In this case, 7th October will be considered as Day Zero as report meets the crieteria of valid report with 4 elements of MSI.

If a CRO which is in contract with a pharma company (manufacturer) for managing its drug safety activities and this CRO receives information about an adverse reaction from a health care professional on 2nd September 2014, then in this case Day Zero will be considered 2nd September 2014 as CRO is in a contract with the manufacturer.

4.15   Database to collect ICSRs

All 'Individual Case Safety Reports' (ICSRs) are entered in the company's safety database and in the regulatory authority's safety database. They are examined individually and in the aggregate for a product in order to identify a potential signal (early warning related to safety concern) or a new risk factor for a reaction to a product, such as a sub-group of patients at particular risk.

In addition to the national regulatory agency databases of spontaneous reports and the company databases, there are two over-arching international databases. They are:

- Vigibase - World Health Organization operates a global scheme involving national collaborating centres (most of the national regulatory agencies worldwide) and a coordinating centre in Sweden - the Uppsala Monitoring Centre (UMC).The UMC database i.e."Vigibase" is the only database in the world that includes all the regulatory authority and company ADR reports. The regulatory authorities send all serious adverse reaction reports that they have received to Vigibase. The UMC has a panel of independent experts who review the data for signals of new adverse reactions. Aggregate data from Vigibase are made available to pharmaceutical companies for purchase.

- EUDRAVIGILANCE safety database - EMA maintains this database. It includes ICSRs received from all companies with products marketed in the European Economic Area, reports received by the national regulatory agencies in the EEA, and serious cases from clinical trials. This database is linked electronically to the national regulatory agency databases. Exchanges of data with national regulatory agency database and with the company databases takes place electronically.

4.16 Overview of reporting adverse event/adverse reaction during clinical trial and during post marketing space

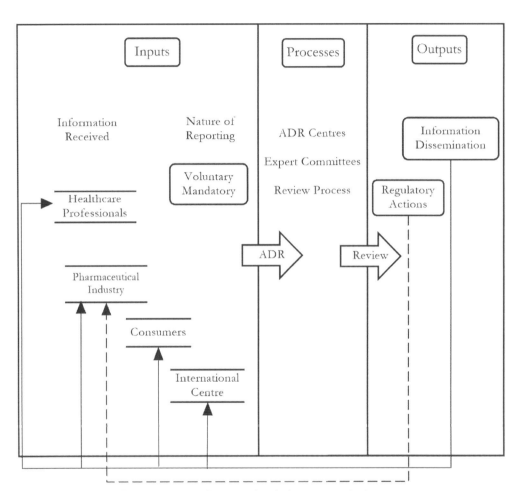

Fig: Adverse reaction reporting during post marketing space

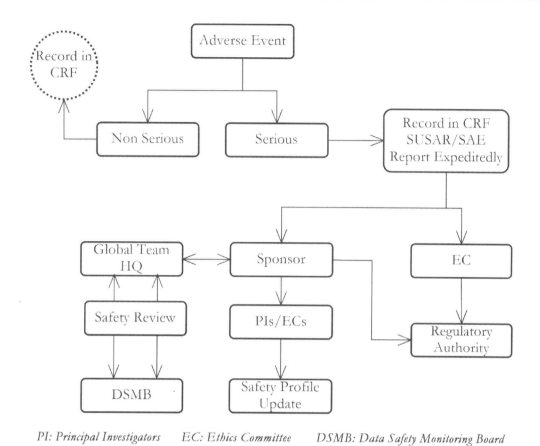

PI: *Principal Investigators*   EC: *Ethics Committee*   DSMB: *Data Safety Monitoring Board*

Fig: Adverse reaction/event reporting during clinical trials

Five

POST MARKETING SURVEILLANCE (PMS)

5.1 Learnings from the chapter

- *Concept and features of PMS*
- *Different methods and sources of PMS*

5.2 Introduction

Once a medicinal product is approved and enters the market, it is available to the general population. So, it is imperative to ensure that the product is safe for general use as this new product is available with limited safety and efficacy information which has been collected in controlled clinical trials (which has a number of limitations like limited number of population, duration etc). Once the drug is available for widespread use, we are able to better evaluate the real safety profile of the drug.

5.3 Post Marketing Surveillance (PMS)

PMS (also known as *post market surveillance*) **is defined as** the practice of monitoring the safety of a medicinal product after it has been released on the market and it is an important part of the science of pharmacovigilance.

5.4 Comparison between pre-marketing trials and PMS

Category	Pre-Marketing Trials	Post Marketing Surveillance
Study phase	Before authorization of medicinal products	Post authorization of medicinal products
Conditions	Carried under standardized conditions	Standardized conditions not present during this phase
Sample Size	Limited/small	Large
Duration	Short/limited	No fixed duration
Study of Low Frequency reactions	Not possible	Possible
Identification of rare and serious ADRs	Less chances	High probability
Exposure to Vulnerable Population	No	Yes

5.5 Features of PMS

PMS is an important tool in PV system due to the features highlighted in the **Fig: Features of PMS**.

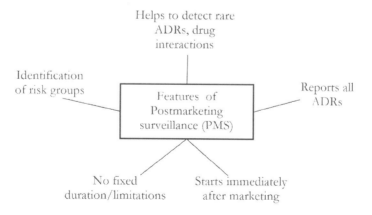

Fig: Features of PMS

5.6   Need of PMS

The primary objective of PMS is to collect more data about the product launched in to the market and to ensure the safe and rational use of product. PMS plays an important role in discovering the undesirable effects related to drug and also collecting additional information on the benefits and risks associated with the drug.

PMS provides:

- Support to study the following:

    - Low frequency reactions (not identified in clinical trials)

    - Long-term effects

    - Drug-drug/food interactions

    - Increased severity and / or reporting frequency of known reactions

- Opportunity to evaluate in unexposed population

- Assessment of cost

5.7   Methods of PMS

PMS may use number of approaches to monitor safety of licensed products. This data is used to assess potential safety signals related to the licensed product. Some of the methods are mentioned in **Fig- Methods of PMS**.

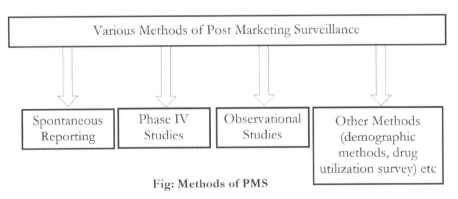

Fig: Methods of PMS

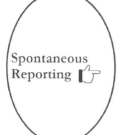

An unsolicited communication by a healthcare professional or a non-healthcare professional to a competent authority, marketing authorization holder or other organization(e.g. regional Pharmacovigilance Centre) that describes one or more suspected adverse reactions in a patient who was given one or more medicinal products and that does not derive from a study or any organized data collection systems.

Fig: Methods of PMS - Spontaneous reporting

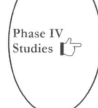

This type of clinical study is done by manufacturers.

This is conducted after the product has gone through phases I, II, III and is already approved for general use.

Purpose of phase IV - assess the safety and side effects of the new drug when it is available to the general population (post launch the medicinal product will be available to a much wider range of patients and under a wider range of conditions than in a controlled clinical trial)

This phase checks whether the product is safe to use over a period of time and that it can be used in other circumstances

Fig: Methods of PMS - Phase IV studies

A type of study in which individuals are observed or certain outcomes are measured. No attempt is made to affect the outcome (for example, no treatment is given).

Examples: Cohort studies, case control studies, cross-sectional studies

Fig: Methods of PMS - Observational studies

5.8 Cohort studies

A defined group of patient (having some specific characteristics "A") is followed up for a defined period of time simultaneously with another group (characterized with absence of characteristic "A") to read the outcome. This study is prospective in nature.

Example: Study is conducted to compare the outcomes of one group which is exposed to smoking habit (smokers) with another group which is not exposed to smoking habit (non-smokers). Both the groups are simply observed (without any interference/intervention) over the time and compared the outcomes (Refer to **Fig - Cohort Studies**).

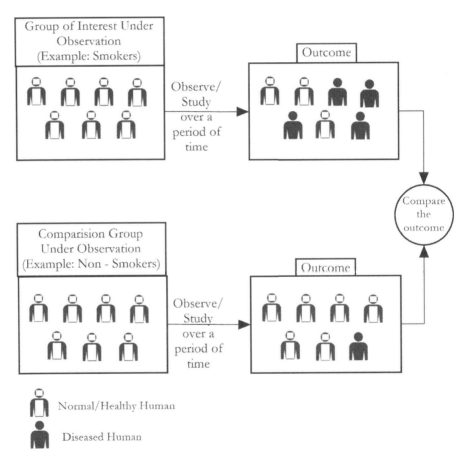

Fig: Cohort Studies

5.9   Case - Control Studies

A study that compares patients who have a disease or outcome of interest (cases) with patients who do not have the disease or outcome (controls), and looks back retrospectively to compare frequency of the exposure to a risk factor for each group to estimate the relationship between the risk factor and the disease. Case control studies are also known as "retrospective studies" and "case-referent studies."

Example: Few cancer patients and non- cancer patients are selected and history of both groups are studied to compare the frequency of exposure to risk factors for each group to estimate the relationship between the risk factor and the disease (Refer to **Fig- Case Control Studies**).

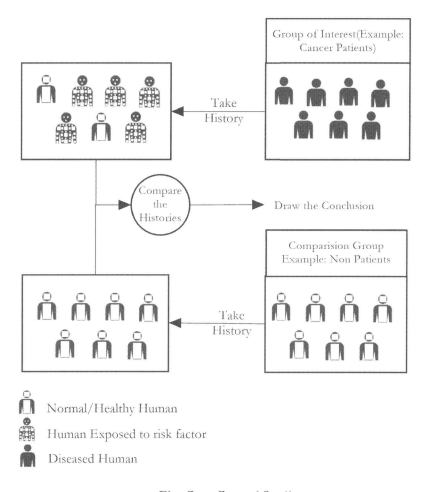

Fig: Case Control Studies

5.10 Cross-Sectional Studies

Cross-sectional study can compare different population groups at a single point in time and also allows to compare many different variables at the same time.

Example: Measure cholesterol levels in daily walkers across two age groups, over 45 and under 45, and compare these to cholesterol levels among non-walkers in the same age groups. However, past or future cholesterol levels are not considered in the study population, only cholesterol levels at one point in time (present) are considered (Refer to **Fig - Cross - sectional Study**).

The cross sectional study is the study for a single point of time (does not consider what happens before and after the study), it does not depict a definite information about cause-effect relationships. Therefore, it is difficult to estimate that daily walking helped to reduce cholesterol levels that were high previously.

In short, the cross-sectional study is done to study prevalence (proportion of a specific population having a particular disease).

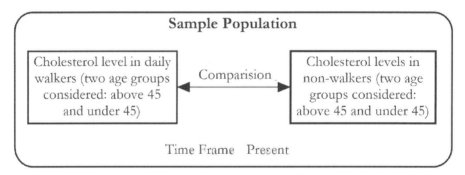

Fig: Cross sectional study

5.11 Sources of Post Marketing Surveillance Report

The PMS reports include study reports as well as spontaneous reports which helps to study the safety profile of a marketed medicinal product. The various sources to obtain PMS reports are depicted in **Fig - Source of Post Marketing Surveillance**.

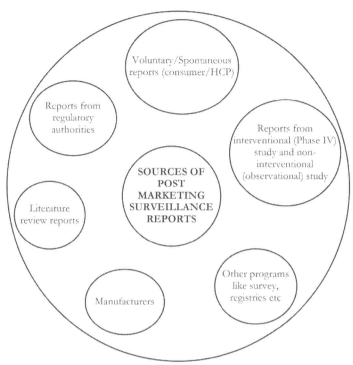

Fig: Sources of Post Marketing Surveillance

Note: For detailed explanation of sources of PMS reports, please refer to CHAPTER 4

5.12   Strengths and Limitations Of Spontaneous Reports

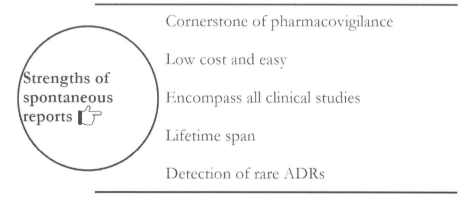

Fig: Strengths of spontaneous reports

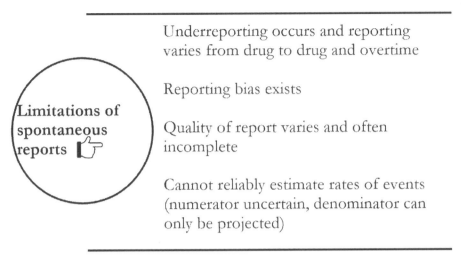

Fig: Limitations of spontaneous reports

5.13   Medium of PMS Reporting

Besides forms, reporter can use telephone, fax, email, internet for reporting adverse effects (Refer to **Fig - Medium of PMS Reporting**).

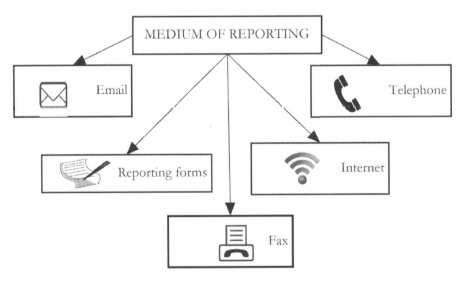

Fig: Medium of PMS reporting

One or more good report can lead to safety signal generation that can be evaluated and the findings can be further communicated. If required, regulatory actions will be also implemented.

Manufactures must establish a PMS for each product.

Well implemented PMS can provide significant benefits:

- Detection of manufacturing problem

- Product quality improvement

- Confirmation of risk analysis

- Knowledge of long term performance or complications

- Customer satisfaction

- Performance in different user population, etc.

Based on information from various sources, the report is prepared which is communicated annually through management review meetings. It also helps to add points to Risk management process and quality management process.

Six

MedDRA

6.1 Learnings from the chapter

- *Need /development of MedDRA and rationale to use MedDRA over other dictionaries*

- *MedDRA structure, conventions and upgradation*

- *MedDRA use and implementation*

- *Description of excluded terms, current/non-current terms, multi-axiality*

- *MSSO details with their organization and services*

6.2 Introduction

Earlier, there was no internationally accepted medical terminology for biopharmaceutical regulatory purposes. Various steps were taken to meet up the requirement, such as: Combination and modification of terminologies were used by many organizations to match up with their requirements. For instance, in Europe, most of the organizations used a combination of the World Health Organization's Adverse Reaction Terminology (WHO-ART©) and the International Classification of Diseases Ninth Revision (ICD-9).

But, all these arrangements had drawbacks listed below:

- Lacked the specificity of terms at the data entry level

- Provided limited data retrieval options

- Did not handle syndromes effectively.

To overcome these deficiencies, organizations developed their own "in-house" terminologies. For example: safety data had frequently been classified for pre-registration clinical trials using ICD terminology and for post-marketing surveillance using COSTART.

These changes lead to problems related to data retrieval, data analysis and cross reference process as different terminologies were used at different stages of product lifecycle.

Furthermore, the use of multiple terminologies in various regions forced the conversion of data from one terminology to another that in turn caused time delays and loss or distortion of data.

In total, these multiple terminology systems made it difficult to manage information exchange among various health related organization and regulators.

In the late 1990s, the International Conference on Harmonization of Technical Requirements for Registration of Pharmaceuticals for Human Use (ICH) developed MedDRA, a rich and highly specific standardized medical terminology to facilitate sharing of regulatory information internationally for medical products used by humans.

Today, the growing use of MedDRA worldwide by regulatory authorities, pharmaceutical companies, clinical research organizations and health care professionals allows better global protection of patient health.

6.3   Development of MedDRA - Chronology

MedDRA was developed using the ICH process by the ICH partners, including WHO. The initial release of MedDRA can be attributed to the chronology listed below:

- **1990** - No standard international medical terminology

- **1993** - Working party of EU regulatory authorities and industry representatives reviewed and amended the UK terminology then called MEDDRA.

- **October 1994** - ICH adopted MEDDRA Version 1.0 as basis for international terminology. An ICH M1 Expert Working Group was formed to further develop the terminology.

- **February 1996** - Version 1.0 was released for alpha testing by pharmaceutical companies and regulatory authorities.

- **July 1997** - ICH agreed to the Version 2.0 and renamed the terminology MedDRA for Medical Dictionary for Regulatory Activities.

- **May 1998** - ICH Steering Committee established the ICH MedDRA Management Board.

- **November 1998** - MedDRA Maintenance and Support Services Organization (MSSO) was contracted to maintain and support MedDRA by IFPMA as a trustee of ICH.

- **January 1999** - Japanese Maintenance Organization (JMO) was established.

- **March 1999** - Initial version of MedDRA (Version 2.1) was available from the MedDRA MSSO and the Japanese version from the JMO.

6.4   MedDRA

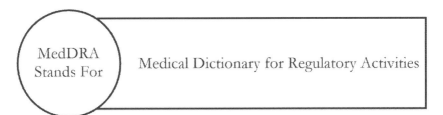

Fig: MedDRA

MedDRA is a clinically-validated international medical terminology used by regulatory authorities and the regulated biopharmaceutical industry. The terminology is used through the entire regulatory process, from pre-marketing to post-marketing phase.

6.5   Objective/ Rationale for MedDRA use over other dictionaries

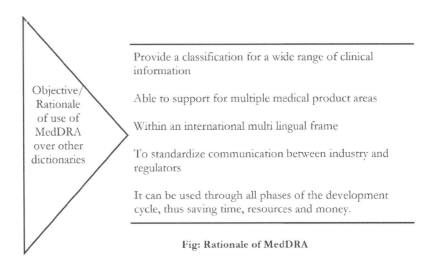

Fig: Rationale of MedDRA

6.6   Benefits of MedDRA

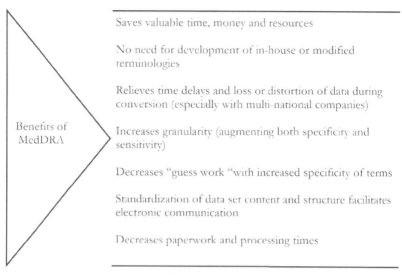

Benefits of MedDRA

Saves valuable time, money and resources

No need for development of in-house or modified terminologies

Relieves time delays and loss or distortion of data during conversion (especially with multi-national companies)

Increases granularity (augmenting both specificity and sensitivity)

Decreases "guess work "with increased specificity of terms

Standardization of data set content and structure facilitates electronic communication

Decreases paperwork and processing times

Fig: Benefits of MedDRA

6.7   Sources of MedDRA terms

Established sources from where the terms have been included in MedDRA

MHRA - Medicines and Healthcare products Regulatory Agency

WHO-ART - World Health Organization Adverse Reaction Terminology

ICD - International Classification of Diseases

ICD-CM - International Classification of Diseases and Clinical Modification

COSTART - Coding Symbols for a Thesaurus of Adverse Reaction Terms

J-ART - Japanese Adverse Reaction Terminology

Fig: MedDRA term sources

6.8 MedDRA is available in several languages

The Japanese translation of MedDRA (MedDRA/J) is maintained by the Japanese Maintenance Organization (JMO) which works with the MSSO to assure that MedDRA/J is kept in synchrony with English MedDRA. The remaining MedDRA translations are centrally maintained by the MSSO (under the direction of the ICH MedDRA Management Board), and changes to English MedDRA are reflected in other languages also.

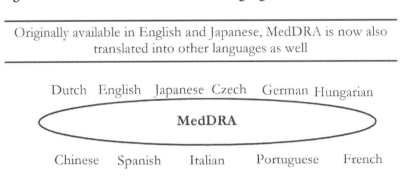

Fig: MedDRA available in several languages

6.9 MedDRA supports electronic submission

ICH developed the electronic Common Technical Document (ICH M8 e CTD) and the electronic Individual Case Safety Report (ICH E2B ICSR) for electronic exchange of data. MedDRA supports the use of these standards which increase the efficiency with which important regulatory information is shared.

e CTD	The CTD is used by pharmaceutical companies to assemble all quality, safety and efficacy information into one format for the submission of new drug applications to ICH regulatory authorities.
ICSR	The ICH E2B standard was developed to support the reporting of ICSRs for both pre- and post-approval periods.

6.10 MSSO: Maintenance and Support Services Organization

MedDRA terminologies must be updated in accordance with changes in regulatory aspects as well as medical/scientific aspects. MSSO services support MedDRA in achieving this objective of evolution in response to medical/scientific advances and changes in the regulatory environment. (Refer to **Fig - MSSO Services to MedDRA**).

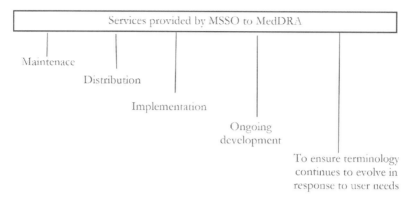

Fig: MSSO Services to MedDRA

6.11   MSSO Governing Body

The activities of Maintenance and Support Services Organization (MSSO) are overseen by an ICH MedDRA Management Board. The MedDRA management board is appointed by the ICH steering committee (Refer to **Fig- MSSO Operations Governed by ICH MedDRA Management Board**).

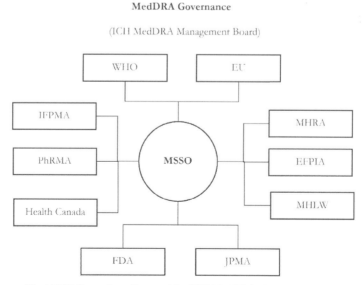

Fig: MSSO Operations Governed by ICH MedDRA Management Board

6.12   MedDRA Upgradations

The MSSO releases updated MedDRA versions twice a year - in March and September. Naming convention for March and September versions as shown in the **fig: MedDRA Upgradation**.

Naming convention for March and September versions are as mentioned below:

-March X.0   -September X.1

X: indicates the number
March version ends with 0
September version ends with 1

Last four versions are listed below:
MedDRA Version 16.0 English March 2013
MedDRA Version 16.1 English September 2013
MedDRA Version 17.0 English March 2014
MedDRA Version 17.1 English September 2014 (current version)

Fig: MedDRA Upgradation

6.13   MedDRA Implementation

MedDRA terminology can be used for data entry, data retrieval, data evaluation and presentation (Refer to **Fig- MedDRA Coding**). MedDRA can be implemented in both pre and post marketing phases of the regulatory process as follows:

- Clinical Studies

- Reports of spontaneous adverse reactions/events

- Regulatory submissions

- Regulated product information

6.14   Scope of MedDRA coding

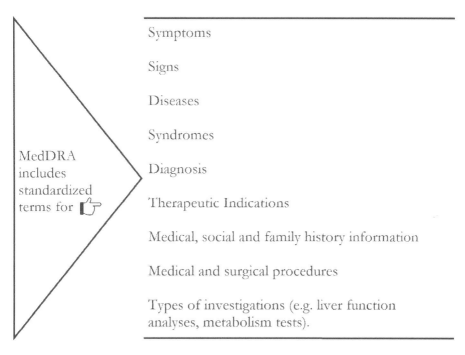

MedDRA includes standardized terms for 👉

Symptoms

Signs

Diseases

Syndromes

Diagnosis

Therapeutic Indications

Medical, social and family history information

Medical and surgical procedures

Types of investigations (e.g. liver function analyses, metabolism tests).

Fig: MedDRA Coding

6.15   MedDRA Structure

Hierarchies are an important mechanism for flexible data retrieval and for the clear presentation of data. The five-level structure of this terminology (Refer to **Fig - MedDRA Structure/Hierarchy**) provides options for retrieving data by specific or broad groupings, according to the level of specificity required. The Lowest Level Term (LLT) level provides maximum specificity.

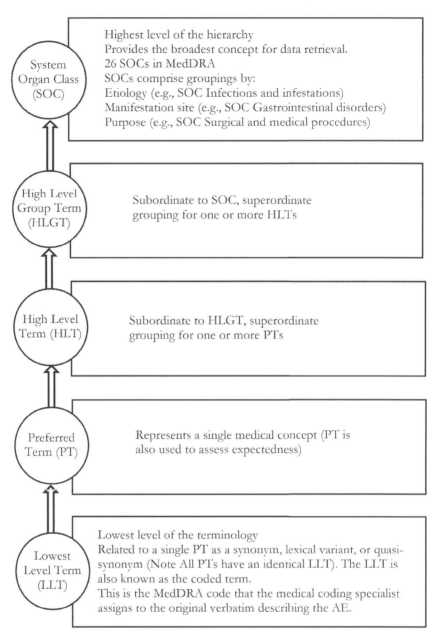

System Organ Class (SOC)
Highest level of the hierarchy
Provides the broadest concept for data retrieval.
26 SOCs in MedDRA
SOCs comprise groupings by:
Etiology (e.g., SOC Infections and infestations)
Manifestation site (e.g., SOC Gastrointestinal disorders)
Purpose (e.g., SOC Surgical and medical procedures)

High Level Group Term (HLGT)
Subordinate to SOC, superordinate grouping for one or more HLTs

High Level Term (HLT)
Subordinate to HLGT, superordinate grouping for one or more PTs

Preferred Term (PT)
Represents a single medical concept (PT is also used to assess expectedness)

Lowest Level Term (LLT)
Lowest level of the terminology
Related to a single PT as a synonym, lexical variant, or quasi-synonym (Note All PTs have an identical LLT). The LLT is also known as the coded term.
This is the MedDRA code that the medical coding specialist assigns to the original verbatim describing the AE.

Fig: MedDRA Structure/Hierarchy

6.16 Example of MedDRA Structure

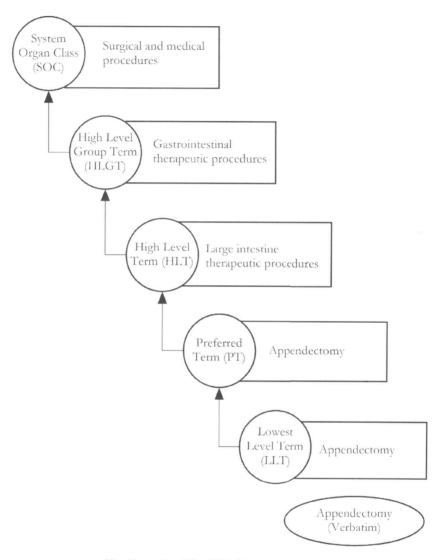

Fig: Example of MedDRA Structure

6.17 LLT relation to PT

LLT is related to single PT as synonym, lexical variant or quasi synonym (Refer to **Fig - LLT Relationship with PT**).

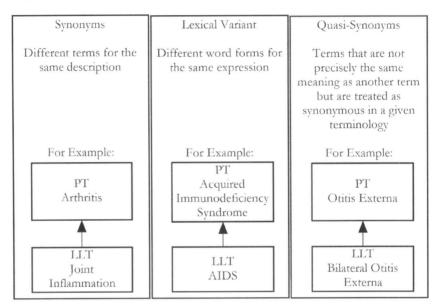

Fig: LLT Relationships with PT

6.18 LLT current and non-current terms

LLTs carry a "**current**" or "**non-current**" flag status. Terms that are very vague, ambiguous, truncated, abbreviated, out-dated or misspelled carry a non-current flag. The terminology retains LLTs with noncurrent flag to preserve historical data for retrieval and analysis. The flag also allows users to implement the terminology within a database and prevent the inadvertent use of non-current LLTs in post-implementation coding.

6.19 Use of MedDRA

There may be many terminologies for the same disease. For e.g investigators can report the headache as "headache", "head pain" or "cephalgia" which will lead to the confusion and duplication of same AE with different terminologies. Therefore a standard terminology is used for coding each AE. This standard terminology coding can be done by using various dictionaries like MedDRA (Medical Dictionary for Regulatory Activities), which will avoid the confusion and duplication.

All MedDRA terms are assigned a unique, 8-digit numeric code. The code is assigned to the translated term in each MedDRA language. This allows for electronic submission of the same concept (e.g., in an Individual Case Safety Report - ICSR) in any of its languages. Codes can fill certain data fields in e-submission types. Benefits of use of codes:

• Codes are comparatively easier to transmit as no language boundaries

• No loss of data

• No mistranslation (by the sender or receiver)

MedDRA was created to assist regulators with sharing information. It is also used by industry, academics, health professionals and other organizations that communicate medical information.

The first use of MedDRA, is in medical coding of any adverse events that occur in the study. This can be done by automatic systems with specialist review or directly by the medical specialist coders. The coder takes the original verbatim describing the adverse event, such as "patient complained about having a headache" and translates it (or codes it) into a standard term, such as simply "headache". This term then is coded to the MedDRA LLT (Low Level Term), such as 10019211 for headache (Refer to **"Fig-Example of Coding Process"**). The safety or pharmacovigilance team review terms and can run queries across all patients based on MedDRA terms or SMQs. At the end of the study, the MedDRA terms are used in the clinical study report to summarize and classify adverse events.

Table: Example of MedDRA Coding

Term	Code
Gastric Hemorrhage (LLT)	10017789
Gastric Haemorrhage (PT)	10017788
Gastric and Oesophageal Haemorrhages (HLT)	10017751
Gastrointestinal Haemorrhages NEC (HLGT)	10017959
Gastrointestinal disorders (SOC)	10017947

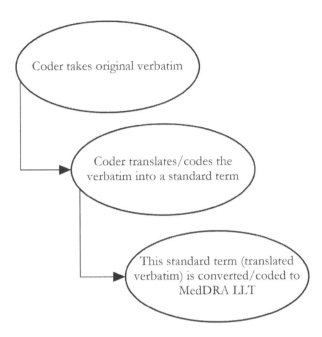

Fig: Example of MedDRA coding process

6.20   Coding examples

Lowest level terms that most accurately reflect the reported verbatim information, should be selected. Only current LLT should be used. Noncurrent LLTs are for legacy conversion/ historical purposes.

Example: "skin rash on face and neck".

If a term contain multiple body sites (for example; skin rash on face and skin rash on neck) and all link to same PT (i.e. rash), the "relevant medical event" should be selected (skin rash on face and neck- "skin rash").

Table: Example - Skin Rash

Reported	LLT Selected	Comment
Skin rash on face and neck	Skin rash	LLT Rash on face, LLT Neck rash and LLT Skin rash All linked to PT Rash

6.21 No scope for either Subtraction or Addition of Information

Table: Term Selection for Diagnosis

Reported	LLT Selected	Comment
Anaphylactic reaction Rash, dysponea, Hypotension, Laryngospasm diagnosis	Anaphylactic reaction	If both a diagnosis and its characteristic sign and symptoms are reported, it is sufficient to select a term for diagnosis

Table: Do not make diagnosis if only signs/symptoms reported

Reported	LLT Selected	Comment
Abdominal pain, increased serum amylase and increased serum lipase	Abdominal pain	It is inappropriate to assign on LLT for diagnosis of "pancreatitis"
	Serum amylase increased	
	Lipase increased	

6.22 MedDRA Conventions

Spellings

British spellings are used at PT and above level while at the LLT level British spellings and American spellings counterpart of the same term are included.
PT and above levels- British Spelling
LLT- British and American Spellings
Example: Under LLT - Diarrhoea / Diarrhea
Under PT and above levels - Diarrhoea.

Capitalization

It can be used for the first letter of each term, proper names and abbreviations.
Example: AIDS

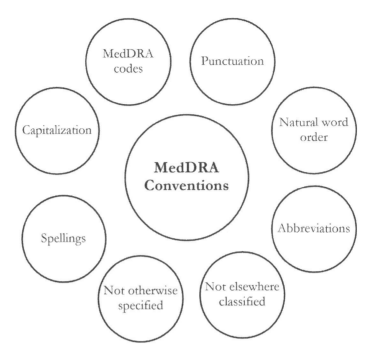

Fig: MedDRA Conventions

Universally accepted abbreviations

It can be found at the LLT level.
Example: HIV (human immunodeficiency virus)
CBC(complete blood count)

Natural word order

It is maintained at the PT level except when reversal of word allows similar terms to be grouped together.
Example: Gastric heamorrhage, Duodenal heamorrhage

Punctuation

It is limited to apostrophes in people's names and some terms.
Example: Glaucoma steroid - induced, Stevens - Johnson syndrome

NOS (Not Otherwise Specified)

"NOS" terms are found at LLT level and are meant to represent concepts for which no further specification is available (eg: during coding of adverse event).Terms carrying "NOS" reflect non specific terms and can only be interpreted with reference to other terms specified in the terminology. For coding, coder should apply most specific terms available(eg: LLT cluster headaches vs. LLT Headache NOS).

NEC (Not Elsewhere Classified)

It is a standard abbreviation used to denote groupings of miscellaneous terms that do not fit into the other hierarchical classifications within a particular SOC (i.e. when terminology does not allow for specificity of reported terms).The "NEC" designation is used with some HLGTs, HLTs, and LLT for grouping purposes. For example : HLT Bladder disorders NEC includes a diverse range of PTs including PT Bladder stenosis, PT Bladder granuloma and PT Bladder telangiectasia.

MedDRA codes

In MedDRA, code refers to eight digit number assigned to each term. These numeric codes are just identification number but not coded information and does not reflect organization of dictionary. A code is assigned to all terms across all categories. Initially, the codes were assigned in alphabetical order starting with 10000001. New terms added to the terminology are assigned the next sequential number. Codes are never reused.

6.23   Multi-Axiality

Definition of Multi-Axiality

Multi Axiality is a characteristic which allows a term to be represented in more than one SOC and to be grouped by different classifications (e.g., by etiology or manifestation site). It has been further explained in the below points:

- Enables retrieval and presentation via different data sets.

- Grouping terms are pre-defined in the terminology and not selected on an ad hoc basis by data entry staff.

- The terminology is structured in such a way that selection of a data entry term leads to automatic assignment of grouping terms higher in the hierarchy.

- Each Preferred Term (PT) is assigned a Primary SOC (however, many PT have a Secondary SOC). A PT can connect to a specific SOC via only one path.
  PT-HLT-HLGT-SOC (1)
  PT-HLT-HLGT-SOC (2)

Example of Multi-Axiality

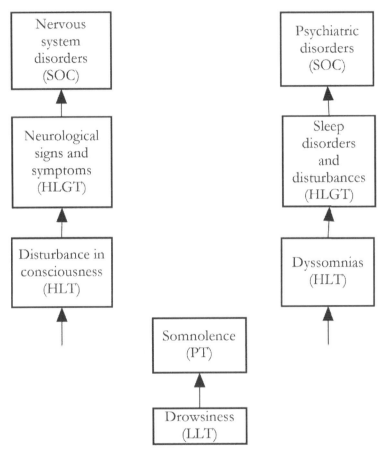

Fig: Example of Multi-Axiality (Primary
SOC - Nervous System Disorders)

Purpose of Primary SOC

- Decrease the risk of double counting of events during cumulative data outputs (secondary SOC can increase the risk)

• It is used to support consistent data presentation for reporting to regulators

Secondary SOCs are used for alternative presentations of data and other type of scientific analysis.

6.24   Excluded Terms

The excluded term refers to the exclusion criteria used in the development of the terminology do not necessarily limit the terminology's expansion scope.

• Since this is a medical terminology, the following terms used in regulatory affairs are out of scope:

  – Equipment/device/diagnostic product terminology

  – Drug/product terminology

  – Study design

  – Demographics (including patient sex, age, race and religion)

• As its focus is on health effects in individual patients, qualifiers that refer to populations rather than individual patients, e.g., rare, frequent are excluded.

• Numerical values associated with laboratory parameters are excluded (e.g. serum sodium 141 mEq/L).

• Descriptors of severity like severe, mild are excluded (with exceptions).

Examples of excluded terms

Table: Example - Excluded Terms

Reported	LLT Selected (for test name)	Comment
Increased blood sugar	Blood Glucose	LLT Blood glucose increased should NOT be selected as it is both a test name and a result*

Table: Example - Excluded Terms

Reported	LLT Selected (for test name)	Comment
Haemoglobin 7.5 gram/dL	Haemoglobin	LLT Haemoglobin decreased should NOT be selected as it is both a test name and a result*

* MedDRA is used only for test names, NOT for test results

6.25   SMQ

SMQ - Standardised MedDRA Queries (SMQs) are tools developed to facilitate retrieval of MedDRA-coded data as a first step in investigating drug safety issues in pharmacovigilance and clinical development. SMQs are validated, pre-determined sets of MedDRA terms grouped together .SMQs have been developed with the CIOMS Working Group on Standardized MedDRA Queries that provides pharmacovigilance expertise and validation of SMQs. The SMQs are maintained with each release of MedDRA by the MSSO.

6.26   SOC Names

The 26 system organ classes are:

- Blood and lymphatic system disorders

- Cardiac disorders

- Congenital, familial and genetic disorders

- Ear and labyrinth disorders

- Endocrine disorders

- Eye disorders

- Gastrointestinal disorders

- General disorders and administration site conditions

- Hepatobiliary disorders

- Immune system disorders

- Infections and infestations

- Injury, poisoning and procedural complications

- Investigations

- Metabolism and nutrition disorders

- Musculoskeletal and connective tissue disorders

- Neoplasms benign, malignant and unspecified (incl cysts and polyps)

- Nervous system disorders

- Pregnancy, puerperium and perinatal conditions

- Psychiatric disorders

- Renal and urinary disorders

- Reproductive system and breast disorders

- Respiratory, thoracic and mediastinal disorders

- Skin and subcutaneous tissue disorders

- Social circumstances

- Surgical and medical procedures

- Vascular disorders.

Seven

CAUSALITY ASSESSMENT

7.1 Learnings from the chapter

- *Introduction to causality assessment*
- *Various methods used for causality assessment*
- *Concept of De-challenge and Re-challenge*

7.2 Introduction

Adverse drug reactions (ADRs) has become one of the prominent reason for hospital admissions, morbidity and mortality of patient as a result of which, the financial burden has increased on individual, society and world economy. To minimize the sufferings of the patients from ADRs, it is essential to establish a causal relationship between the drug and the events. This is done through causality assessment.

7.3 Causality Assessment

By definition, causality assessment is the evaluation of the likelihood that a particular treatment is the cause of an observed adverse event. It assesses the relationship between a drug treatment and the occurrence of an adverse event.

Causality assessment is an integral part of pharmacovigilance, contributing to better evaluation of the risk-benefit profiles of medicines and is an essential part of evaluating ADR reports in early warning systems and for regulatory purposes.

7.4 Methods of Causality Assessment

There are a number of methods ranging from short questionnaires to comprehensive algorithms for causality assessment of ADRs with various advantages and disadvantages. So far, no ADR causality assessment method has shown consistent and reproducible measurement of causality; therefore, no single method is universally accepted. Three broad categories of various methods of causality assessment have been depicted in the **fig: Methods of Causality Assessment**.

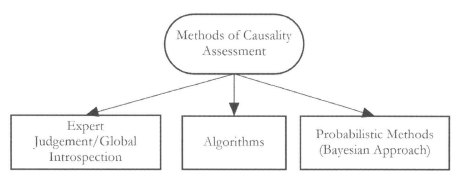

Fig: Methods of Causality Assessment

Expert Judgement/Global Introspection

This method is most commonly used by clinicians

Individual assessments based on previous knowledge and experience in the relevent field

Standardized tools are not used in this method

Limitations of this method
Lacks transparancy
Difference in Human Judgement leads to inconsistencies

Fig: Global Introspection

Probabilistic Methods (Bayesian Approach)

This approach uses specific findings in a case to transform the prior estimate of probability into a posterior estimate of probability of drug causation.

Prior Probability is calculated from epidemiological information and pre-marketing clinical trials

Posterior probabiity combines this background information with the evidence in the individual case to come up with an estimate of causation.

Fig: Probabilistic Methods

Algorithms

Algorithms

Set of specific questions with associated scores for calculating the likelihood of a cause-effect relationship.

Structured and standardized method of assessment

Advantages of Algorithms: Transparency & consistency

Limitations of Algorithms: Decreased ability to apply the clinical judgement.

No single algorithm is universally accepted.

Fig: Algorithms

Lots of algorithms have been developed. Some examples of algorithms/scales used for causality assessment have been shown in the **fig: Algorithm names**.

7.5   Algorithm Names

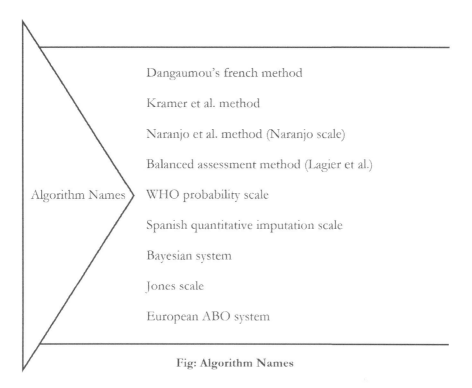

Algorithm Names

Dangaumou's french method

Kramer et al. method

Naranjo et al. method (Naranjo scale)

Balanced assessment method (Lagier et al.)

WHO probability scale

Spanish quantitative imputation scale

Bayesian system

Jones scale

European ABO system

Fig: Algorithm Names

Causality assessment algorithms differ in many respects but share certain common features.

- Questions are used to capture details of the ADR

- Different procedures are thereafter adopted to convert answers from these questions to estimate probability

7.6   Parameters used in Algorithm Method

Algorithms give structured and standardized methods of assessment in a systematic approach to identify ADRs based on parameters shown in the **fig: Few parameters of algorithm**.

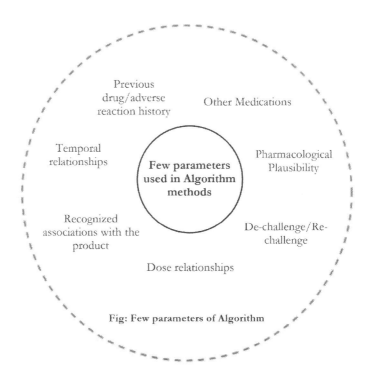

Fig: Few parameters of Algorithm

7.7 Widely Accepted Algorithms

Although there are a number of algorithms developed to assess causality between drug and the event, but most widely accepted algorithms are WHO Scale and Naranjo Scale.

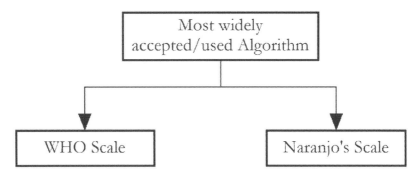

Fig: Widely Accepted Algorithm

7.8   WHO Scale

The level of causal association is groped into six categories which are based on the criteria (number of criteria being met) mentioned in the **fig: criteria of WHO scale**.

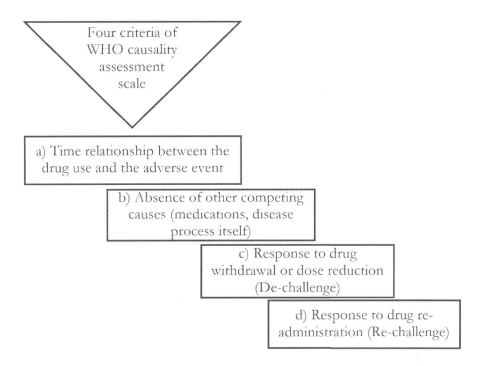

Fig: Criteria of WHO Scale

WHO -causality assessment method
Causal category is "certain" when all the four criteria are met.
Causal category is "probable" when criteria a, b and c are met.
Causal category is "possible" when only criterion a is met.
Causal category is "unlikely" when criteria a and b are not met.

Beside these four categories, ADR can also be categorized into "Unclassified/Conditional" or "Unassessable/Unclassifiable" in WHO-UMC causality assessment. The term "Unclassified/Conditional" is applied when more data is needed and such data is being sought or is already under examination. Finally when the information in a report is incomplete or contradictory and cannot be complemented or verified, the verdict is "Unclassifiable". This has been explained in the tabular form shown below:

Categories	Time sequence	Other drugs/disease ruled out-	Dechallenge	Rechallenge
Certain	Yes	Yes	Yes	Yes
Probable	Yes	Yes	Yes	No
Possible	Yes	No	No	No
Unlikely	No	No	No	No

7.9   Naranjo Scale

Question	Yes	No	Don't know
Are there previous conclusion reports on this reaction?	+1	0	0
Did the adverse event appear after the suspect drug was administered?	+2	-1	0
Did the AR improve when the drug was discontinued or a specific antagonist was administered?	+1	0	0
Did the AR reappear when drug was re-administered?	+2	-1	0
Are there alternate causes [other than the suspect drug] that could solely have caused the reaction?	-1	+2	0
Did the reaction reappear when a placebo was given?	-1	+1	0

Was the drug detected in the blood [or other fluids] in a concentration known to be toxic?	+1	0	0
Was the reaction more severe when the dose was increased or less severe when the dose was decreased?	+1	0	0
Did the patient have a similar reaction to the same or similar drugs in any previous exposure?	+1	0	0
Was the adverse event confirmed by objective evidence?	+1	0	0
Scoring for Naranjo algorithm: >9 = definite ADR; 5–8 = probable ADR; 1–4 = possible ADR; 0 = doubtful ADR.			

7.10   Challenge

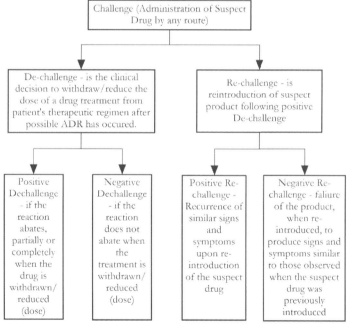

Fig: De-Challenge & Re-Challenge

Eight

SIGNAL MANAGEMENT PROCESS

8.1 Learnings from the chapter

- *Concept of Signal and sources of Signal*

- *Signal Management Process Overview in detail which includes signal detection, validation, strengthening, assessment, prioritization, evaluation and decision making*

8.2 Introduction

The safety data generated during clinical trials is always not enough to rule out all possible adverse effect of the drug as the clinical trials have several limitations.

The major limitations of clinical trials:

- Selected and limited number of patients are exposed

- Limited time frame

- Controlled environment

- Limited duration of drug exposure, etc.

To detect rare ADRs, large sample size is required which is not possible in a controlled clinical trial environment. Limitations of clinical trials lead to detection of only more common ADRs. Rough estimation of the power to detect adverse events is generally calculated by "rule of 3" For example, to find out the incidence of 1 in 10,000 at least 30,000 people need to be treated with a drug. To detect the incidence of 1 in 100,000, we can imagine the sample size, which are almost beyond the scope of clinical trials. This in turn suggests that the safety information available even by the well-designed clinical trials is not adequate to answer the safety concern.

Signal is a potential and established indicator of new ADR. Signal is referred as any new possible causal link between a suspected ADR and drug; which was previously unknown or not completely documented.

The primary function of Pharmacovigilance is to ensure the provision of early warnings (signals) with regards to previously unknown adverse effects of medicines. So, with each introduction of a potent new drug, pharmaceutical firm must detect adverse reactions quickly in order to ensure patient safety, minimise costs, protect their brand name and ease regulatory compliance.

8.3   Definition of Signal

WHO Definition of Signal is: "Reported information on a possible causal association between an adverse event and a drug, the relationship being unclear or incompletely documented previously".
Note: A signal is not a confirmatory finding but it is a hypothesis-generating situation that must be validated or disapproved.

8.4   Sources of Signals

Where to find the signals from? This was an issue earlier, but spontaneous reporting system and automation technology has solved this problem as it covers large population and these huge data reservoir contain a multitude of potential signals. Some of the important sources are mentioned in **fig-Sources of Signals**:

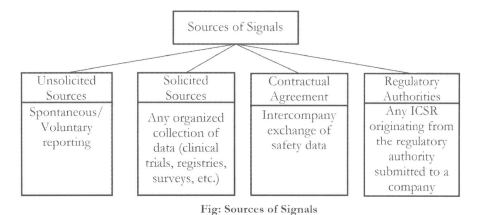

Fig: Sources of Signals

Note: For detailed explanation of sources of signals, please refer to CHAPTER 4

8.5   Signal Management Process

Signal management process refers to "set of activities performed to determine whether there are new risks associated with an active substance or medical product or whether the risk have changed". (Refer to **Fig - Signal Management Process summarized**)

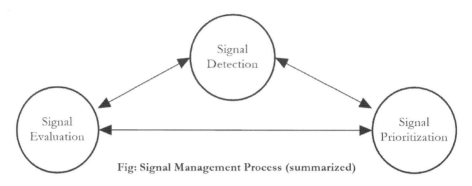

Fig: Signal Management Process (summarized)

8.6   Signal Detection

The act of looking for and/or identifying signals using event data from any source.

Importance of Signal Detection

Importance of Signal Detection

Signal detection is one of the most important objective of Pharmacovigilance. The whole process of risk/benefit evaluation depends on effective detection of signals.

Early signal detection can help in identifying potential risks associated with marketed drugs and the identified risks can be managed effectively which in turn helps the company to protect their brand and provide consumers improved drug.

Continuous monitoring of the risk profile associated with a medicinal product is a legal obligation (including written documentation of this process).

Fig: Importance of Signal Detection

Speed of Signal Detection

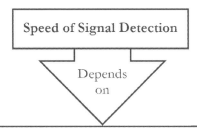

Fig: Speed of Signal Detection

Factors favouring and hindering signal detection

The connection between a drug and an adverse effect is often difficult to detect. Signal is basically a clue which points towards a possible relation of ADR with a drug. There are a number of factors which enhance the possibility of finding such a clue and similarly, there are a number of factors which hinder the possibility of finding such a clue. Some factors are mentioned in **Fig - Factors favouring Signal detection and Factors hindering Signal detection.**

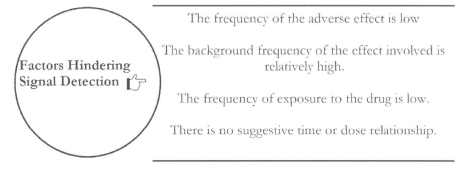

Fig: Factors hindering signal detection

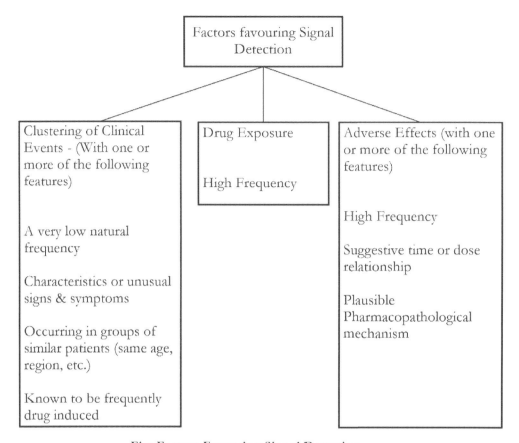

Fig: Factors Favouring Signal Detection

Signal Detection Methods

Signal detection is a process of identification of relation between drug and adverse event/reaction. Careful judgment and analysis on the ground of chemical, pharmacological and therapeutic point of view is necessary to establish the association. Unknown ADR, strong statistical connection, serious but unlabelled, low background noise, high potential relevance are the positive indicator of the signal.

Signals have qualitative and quantitative aspects. Different categories of adverse effects need different methods of detection.

The number of reports needed to provide sufficient evidence for a signal may differ depending upon the nature of effect, quality of report and possible evidence from other sources.

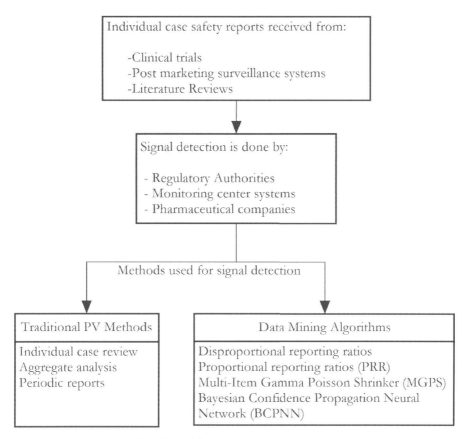

Fig: Signal Detection Methods

A single good report (e.g. with a positive rechallenge) may be a valid signal.

When there are a relatively small number of cases, pharmacovigilance professionals can review the data, focusing on clinical characteristics of individual cases. Statistical and epidemiological methods would be useful to summarize a large amount of data. (The large amount of data, however, does not preclude the importance of clinical judgment and assessment.) So, in addition to the traditional hands-on review of spontaneous cases and other safety information by trained medical personnel, "data mining" may also be carried out (Refer to **Fig - Signal Detection Methods**). This is the process of applying sophisticated statistical algorithms to large safety databases to determine whether certain adverse events (AEs) are being reported for a medicine with a greater frequency than expected (i.e., a signal of disproportionate reporting, or SDR), based on a statistical model.

Data mining methods are based on the concept of disproportionality. It is assumed that in the absence of disproportionality, the distributions of reported adverse events are the same across drugs. If a specific adverse event were associated with a given drug and this event would have higher reporting frequency then it creates reporting disproportionality. Statistic of disproportionate reporting are screened based on the ranking of drug-event combination by the level of disproportionality, or statistical "unexpectedness." Disproportionality analysis i the most commonly used method. This analysis involves the "2x2" contingency table, which classifies report according to the presence or absence of the suspect drug of interest and the presence or absence of the event of interest in reports. It measures the association in terms o relative reporting (RR), proportional reporting rate ratio (PRR), reporting odds ratio (ROR and information component (IC).

Contingency Table

	Event of Interest	All Other Events	Total
Product of Interest	A	B	A+B
All Other Products	C	D	C+D
Total	A+C	B+D	A+B+C+D

All measures of disproportionate reporting are basically calculation of (observed/expected frequency. In PV, the expected data is also referred to as "background" frequency.

For example, a score can be generated for a particular AE-medicine combination (e.g. frequency of bleeding disorder with Drug X) and compared with the score for all medicine in the database (i.e., frequency of bleeding disorder across all medicines). When the AE-Drug X score is greater than the AE-all medicine score, a safety signal may have been detected, depending on the clinical context.

Other available tools (varying in degrees of development) include regression analysis clustering, link analysis, deviation detection, and neural networks. These quantitative methodologies go beyond basic signal detection to assess patterns, time trends, and event associated with more complex phenomena such as drug-drug interactions, which may be more difficult to link by manual review. It is crucial to remember that, no matter how sophisticated the statistical and quantitative tools that are available, qualitative medical review and assessmen are necessary to guide the quantitative analysis and evaluation.

8.7   Signal Validation

Signal validation is the process of evaluating the data supporting the detected signal in order to verify whether they are real or not. Often, an apparent signal can result just from the disease that the drug is treating - so if a drug is used in patients for the treatment of high blood pressure, it would not be surprising to find reports of high blood pressure itself, and also kidney disease, stroke and heart failure, because these are either contributory or complications of high blood pressure. Various ways to validate a signal is mentioned in **Fig - Signal Validation**.

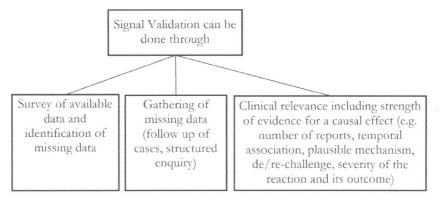

Fig: Signal Validation

Signal becomes validated if the verification of all relevant documentation is suggestive of a new potentially causal association, or a new aspect of a known association, and therefore justifies further assessment of the signal.

8.8   Signal Strengthening

Once the signal is detected and validated, it is strengthen by available evidence. Signal strengthening is the process of making signal more evidence based and reliable. This is done through seeking information from different sources (refer to **Fig - Signal Strengthening**).

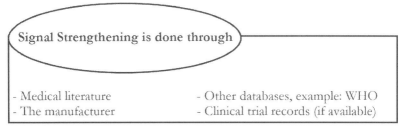

Fig: Signal Strengthening

Analogy is done with other related drugs. Absence of supporting data doesn't imply false signal.

8.9 Signal Assessment

Signal assessment consists of a thorough pharmacological, medical and epidemiological assessment of all the information available on the signal of interest.

Objective of Signal assessment

Objectives of Signal Assessment

To examine the evidence for a causal association between an adverse reaction and a suspected medicinal product

To quantify this association (preferably in absolute terms)

To identify the need for additional data collection or for any regulatory action

Fig: Signal Assessment

Criteria of Signal assessment

Criteria	Explanation
Quantitative	
Strength of the Association	The number of case reports (in relation to exposure to the drugs), statistical disproportionality & significance
Qualitative	
Consistency of the data	The general presence of characteristic feature or pattern, and absence or rarity of converse findings
Exposure Response Relationship	Site, timing, dosage-response relationship, reversibility
Biological Plausibility of the hypothesis	Pharmacological & Pathological Mechanism
Experimental Findings	Rechallange, drug dependent antibodies, high blood or tissue concentrations, abnormal metabolites, diagnostic markers
Analogy	Previous experience with related drugs, event known to frequently be drug induced
Nature & Quality of the data	Characteristic nature & objectivity of the event, accuracy & validity of documentation, case causality assessment.

8.10 Signal Prioritization

A key element of the signal management process is to promptly identify signals with important public health impact or that may affect the benefit-risk balance of the medicinal product in treated patients. These signals require urgent attention and need to be evaluated without delay. This prioritization process should consider the strength and consistency of the evidence, e.g., a high number of valid cases reported in a short Period of time, identification of the signal in different settings (e.g. general practice and hospital).

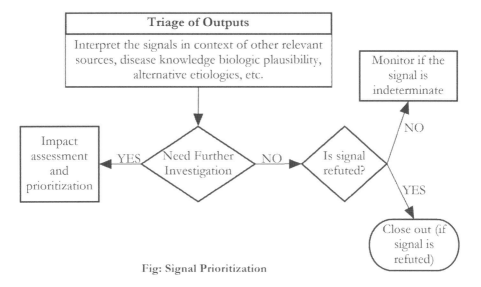

Fig: Signal Prioritization

Categorization of Signal

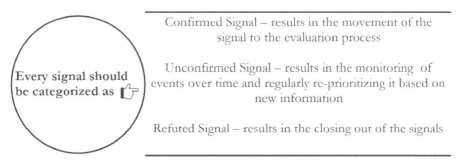

Fig: Signal Categorization

Methods of Signal Prioritization

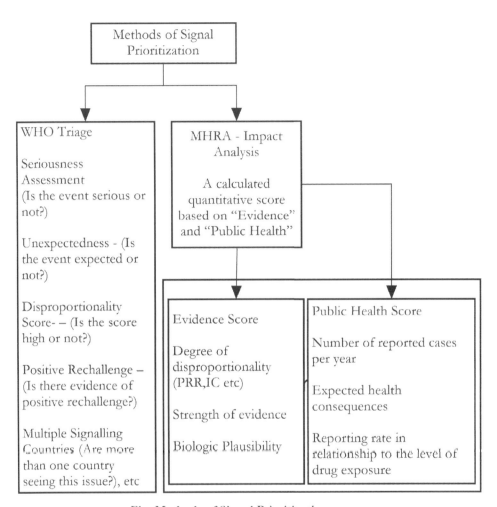

Fig: Methods of Signal Prioritization

8.11   Signal Evaluation

The information collected in the signal evaluation process is intimately tied to risk identification and may result into the feeding of the signal into the risk management planning processes.

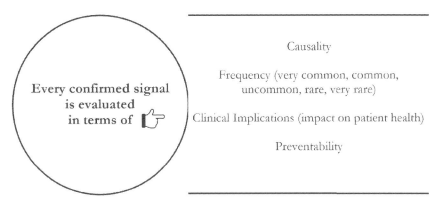

Fig: Signal Evaluation

8.12   Decision making

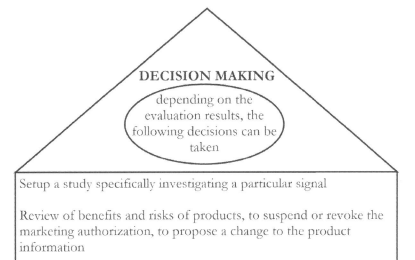

Fig: Decision Making

8.13   Signal Management Process-detailed

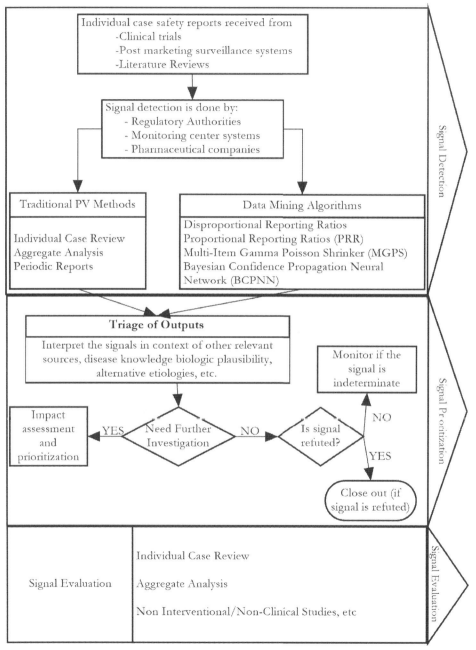

Fig: Signal Management Process - Detailed

Nine

RISK MANAGEMENT PLAN

9.1 Learnings from the chapter

- *Need of risk management*

- *Concept of Risk management system*

- *Detail description of RMP including components, element, purpose and preparation period*

- *REMS basics and comparison of REMS with RMP*

9.2 Introduction

To ensure the safety of drugs, it is essential to assess the measures taken for appropriate management of the risks associated with drugs at any time from the development phase to the regulatory review and the post-marketing phase.

9.3 Risks associated with medicinal products

Along with the therapeutic value, the medicinal products may have certain risks (as depicted in the **fig: Sources of Risk from Medicinal Products**)

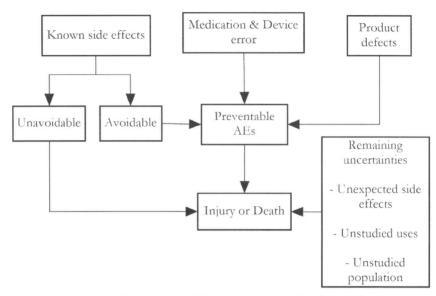

Fig: Sources of Risk from Medicinal Products

9.4   Risk management system

Definition of Risk management system

Risk management system is a set of activities and interventions designed to identify, characterize prevent or minimize risks relating to medicinal product, including the assessment of the effectiveness of those activities and interventions.

When a new medicinal product is marketed, the manufacturer/MAH must ensure that the benefits associated with the concerned medicinal product outweighs the risks by a good margin

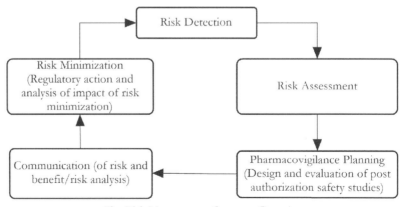

Fig: Risk Management System - Overview

Risk management system is a continuous process of minimizing product's risks throughout its lifecycle in order to ensure that benefit of a particular product exceeds risks. To achieve this, activities and interventions are deployed to a drug to manage and mitigate known and possible risks, with the aim of protecting the individuals.

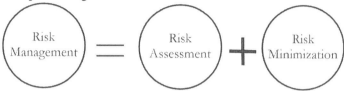

Fig: Risk Management

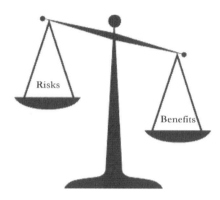

9.5   Need for Risk Management

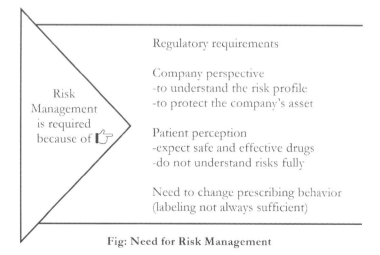

Fig: Need for Risk Management

9.6   Risk management plan (RMP)

Risk management plan is a detailed description of risk management system. It is a regulatory document submitted to the Health authorities. RMP may be required any time after commercialization of product, when safety concern has emerged.

9.7   Purpose of the Risk Management Plan (RMP)

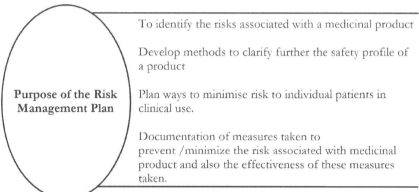

Purpose of the Risk Management Plan

To identify the risks associated with a medicinal product

Develop methods to clarify further the safety profile of a product

Plan ways to minimise risk to individual patients in clinical use.

Documentation of measures taken to prevent /minimize the risk associated with medicinal product and also the effectiveness of these measures taken.

Fig: Purpose of Risk Management

9.8   Basic Components of a Risk Management Plan

The RMP consists of the following three elements for individual drugs (refer to **fig Components of RMP**):

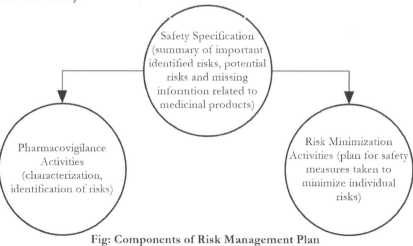

Safety Specification (summary of important identified risks, potential risks and missing informtion related to medicinal products)

Pharmacovigilance Activities (characterization, identification of risks)

Risk Minimization Activities (plan for safety measures taken to minimize individual risks)

Fig: Components of Risk Management Plan

9.9   Safety specification

Characterization/Synopsis of the safety profile of the medicinal product including what is known and not known. Safety specification will form the basis of pharmacovigilance plan and the risk minimization plan.

Safety Specifications Include:

Summary of important identified risks of the medicine, potential risks, and missing information.

This summary incorporates the safety profile of the medicine during its life-cycle, either during preclinical testing/pre-approval clinical development or post-approval.

9.10   Pharmacovigilance Activities

Activities for collecting information which are performed in post-marketing. Pharmacovigilance activities are planned to characterize risks, identify new risks, increase the knowledge in general about the safety profile of the medicinal product.

Pharmacovigilance Activities Include:

Active surveillance (e.g., medical records reviews, patient or physician interviews, prescription event monitoring, data from registries).

Epidemiology studies (retrospective or prospective).

Further clinical studies (specific safety studies, larger studies over longer periods).

Drug utilization studies (which describe how a drug is marketed, prescribed, and used in a specified population—often stratified by age, gender, concomitant medications, etc—and how these factors influence clinical, social, and economic outcomes).

9.11   Risk minimization activities

Planning and implementation of risk minimization and mitigation activities and the assessmen of the effectiveness of these activities. Activities for safety measures taken to minimize the risks

---

Risk Minimization Activities Include:

Provision of information and education for healthcare professionals

Additional educational material about the medicine and its use (patient information brochures, visual aids, physician prescribing guides/checklists, pharmacist dispensing guides/checklists).

Training programs (patient- or physician-oriented)

Restricted use of the medicine (e.g. for use/dispensing only in hospital, or where specific equipment is available), etc.

With regard to Pharmacovigilance and risk minimization activities, there are two types o activities:

- **Routine activities** - Routine activities are the activities conducted for all drug by Marketing Authorization Holders (MAHs), specifically collecting information o adverse drug reactions and information provision by package inserts of drugs, etc.

- **Additional activities** - These activities are conducted individually based on th individual properties, such as early post-marketing phase vigilance of new drugs or use results surveys post-marketing clinical studies and distribution of materials to ensure th proper use of drugs that require caution, etc.

9.12   Elements of RMP

The various aspects covered under RMP are depicted in the **fig: elements of RMP**.

9.13   When to Prepare RMP

Once RMP is approved by health authorities, Market Authorization Holder (MAH) has legal obligation to perform activities described in RMP. RMP preparation can be required i different situations described in the **fig :When to prepare RMP**.

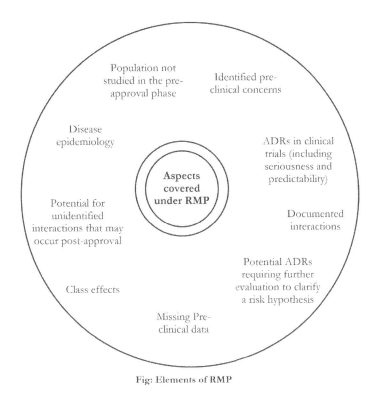

Fig: Elements of RMP

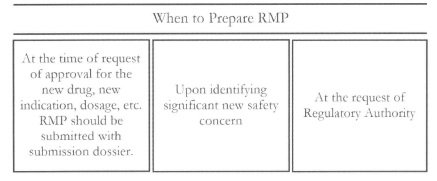

Fig: When to prepare RMP

Monitoring safety of drug after commercialization is always paramount as it is related to human well being. An effective risk management requires measurable objectives. Evaluation of risk minimization strategy for a product should be done in terms of outcomes and not only its individual elements i.e. scope includes routine and additional risk minimization measures. If risk minimization is not working , need to find out the reasons for failure whether it is due to implementation defect or conceptual issue is there. Drug utilization studies play an important role as information of these studies are less biased than survey results. Proposal need to be feasible, realistic and underpinned by science. RMP needs to be integrated with pharmacovigilance planning, PSUR, etc.

9.14   Risk Evaluation and Mitigation Strategy (REMS)

Risk Evaluation and Mitigation
Strategy (REMS)

REMS ensure that the benefits of a medicine outweigh its risks.

REMS may be required by the FDA as part of the approval process for a new product, or for an approved product when new safety information emerges. An applicant may also voluntarily submit a REMS.

REMS is a strategy to manage a known or potential serious risk associated with a medicine.

Its purpose is to allow patients continued access to certain medicines for which there are safety concerns that may be managed through appropriate use.

REMS may also include one or more of:
  •A Medication Guide.
  •A patient package insert.
  •A communication plan to disseminate information to health care providers in support of the strategy.
   •Elements to Assure Safe Use of the product, such as:
   - Special training or certification for health care professionals who prescribe or dispense the medicine.
   - Dispensing the medicine only in certain settings (e.g., in a hospital) or with evidence of safe use conditions (e.g., laboratory test results).
   - Monitoring or registration of each patient using the medicine.

An implementation system for certain elements to ensure safe use.

9.15 Comparison between RMP and REMS

RMP	REMS
RMP – Risk Management Plan	REMS – Risk Evaluation & Mitigation Strategy
Required by – EU and other countries	Needed by FDA
For every product	For some products
Management of overall assessment of risk during the life of product	Management of Risk Minimization of specific identified risk during life of the product.
Elements of RMP – safety specification, pharmacovigilance plan, risk minimization plan	Elements of REMS - Medication Guide, Communication Plan, Elements to assure safe use (ETASU).

Ten

10.1   Learnings from the chapter

- *Concept of Labeling with features and importance*

- *Definitions of expected/unexpected ADR/ADE*

- *Details of conditions to determine an event/reaction unexpected*

- *Details of assessment criteria of expectedness*

10.2   Introduction

Labeling is the process or obligation of including information to accompany a medicinal product. In general, labeling includes the name of the drug and details of any adverse events, contradictions, etc. With more and more products in the market, product labeling is growing in importance daily. Normally, labeling is referred to vial and carton labels and any insert (direction for use, etc) included with a drug product, biological product, medical device.

10.3   Labeling

Definition of Labeling

In the USA, FDA defines labeling as "all labels and other written, printed, or graphic matter upon any article or any of its containers or wrappers or accompanying such article. All labeling particulars must be consistent with the relevant product license/marketing authorization. The product's particulars must be clearly written on the outer packaging or the immediate packaging (if no outer packaging is present).

10.4   Usual Sections in Labeling

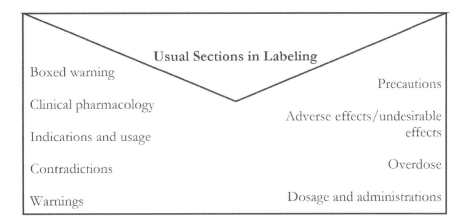

Fig: Sections in Labeling

10.5   Key Features/Importance of Labeling

Key Features/Importance of Labeling			
Provide Basic Information	Instructions for Use	Warning & Contradictions	Minimum Safety Information
Labeling should provide basic information like brand name, the price, the standard certification or expiry date for the products, the name, address of the manufacturer, ingredients, batch no etc.	Label helps to figure out consumption instructions (eg:swallowing, chewing), instruction on storage and maintenance of the product.	A good label should contain warning of possible dangers and hazards. In case of food and medicnies, the labels should provide contradictions and possible side effects.	Labeling can help in reporting about any ADR experienced by any person by giving the data/information about the product, for eg: product name, dosage etc

Fig: Importance of Labeling

10.6   Unexpected/Expected Adverse Drug Event/Reaction

Unexpected Adverse Event/Reaction

An unexpected adverse event/adverse reaction is an ADR whose nature, severity, specificity, or outcome is not consistent with the term or description used in the following documents :

The applicable product information

Current Investigator's Brochure

With the risk information described in the investigational plan

Current labeling of the product

Fig: Unexpected Adverse Events

Expected Adverse Event/Reaction

Events that have been observed previously with the drug administered in humans and documented in the RSI (reference safety information) document.   (Refer to **fig: RSI Document**)

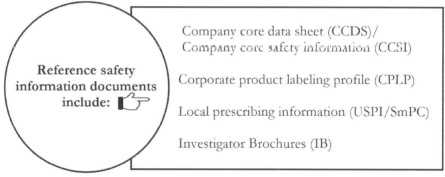

Reference safety information documents include:

Company core data sheet (CCDS)/
Company core safety information (CCSI)

Corporate product labeling profile (CPLP)

Local prescribing information (USPI/SmPC)

Investigator Brochures (IB)

Fig: RSI Documents

NOTE: The term "listedness" is not applicable to expedited reporting but should be used to characterize the ADR according to the Company Core Safety Information. Listedness is based on CCSI which is the core safety information for the molecule available with Marketing Authorization Holder. Expectedness is based on the local document i.e. SmPC, USPI.

10.7   Conditions to consider an event/reaction "Unexpected"

- An adverse event/reaction can be considered unexpected from the perspective of previous observation, not on the basis of what might be anticipated from the pharmacological properties of a medicinal product.

  - Example - Antibiotic A develops gastric issues on intake but it's not necessary that Antibiotic B will produce same issue (unless mentioned) on consumption.

- Any event that is previously not known or anticipated to result from an underlying disease/disorder/condition of the human subject/study population, may also be considered as unexpected event (or any event/reaction which occurs in the course of disease progression).

  - Example: A patient suffering from diarrhea ends up in suffering from dehydration as well. In this case, dehydration is an unexpected event as it occurs in the course of disease progression.

- Reported event/reaction that add significant information on severity, specificity of a known/already documented serious adverse event/ADR is considered unexpected.

- Class labeling - Adverse events listed as occurring with a class of drug or biological product but not specifically mentioned with a particular drug or biological product are considered unexpected.

  - Example, rashes appearing on consuming the antibiotic X would be considered unlabeled/unexpected even though the labeling says "rash may be associated with antibiotics". This is because the said labeling does not specifically state that rash is associated with antibiotic X.

10.8   Criteria for assessing expectedness

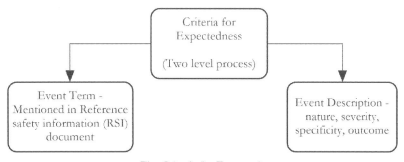

Fig: Criteria for Expectedness

10.9   Severity of Events

If reported event is more severe than the labeled event, then it should be considered unlabeled/unexpected.

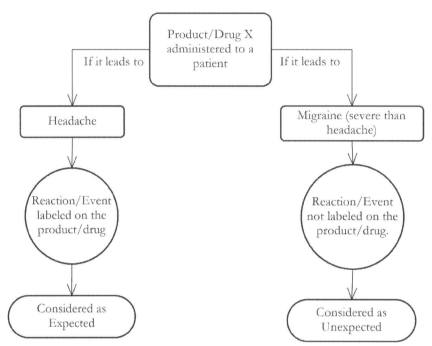

Fig: Example - Severity of Events

Migraine would be unexpected event (by the virtue of greater severity), if only headache is documented in the relevant source document.

10.10   Specificity of Events

A single diagnosis should be considered unexpected if only the broader diagnosis is in the label without the subtypes being mentioned.

Cerebral thromboembolism would be unexpected event (by virtue of greater specificity), if the cerebral vascular accident is documented in the relevant source document.

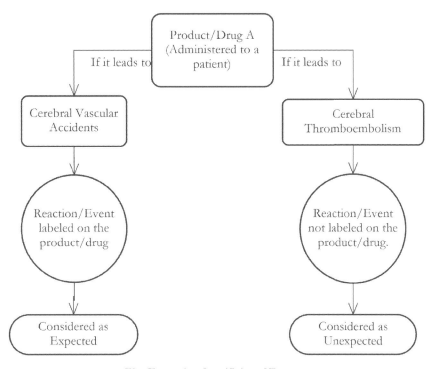

Fig: Example - Specificity of Events

10.11   Outcome

Fatal outcome - unless death is explicitly mentioned in the product information, it should be considered as an unexpected event. Reports of death from an adverse event are considered unlabeled/unexpected unless the possibility of fatal outcome from the adverse event is stated in the labeling.

10.12   Event Term - Signs and Symptoms

If the diagnosis is an expected event, then the sign and symptoms which comprise the diagnosis are also expected. But the reverse is not true.
For example: if the diagnosis (diabetes) is an expected event, then the sign and symptoms (excessive thirst and increased hunger) of diabetes are also expected, but the reverse is not true.

In assessing a case report, medical judgment must be used along with knowledge of regulations if there is any doubt consider the adverse effect as unexpected.

Eleven

PSUR/PBRER

11.1   Learnings from the chapter

- *Detail description of PSUR/PBRER*

- *Timelines for PSUR/PBRER submission*

- *General principles of PBRER*

- *Concept of different birth dates and DSUR basics*

11.2   Introduction

The limitations due to controlled environment of clinical trials make it imperative for the manufacturers and health authorities to continue collection and analysis of data related to medicinal product even post authorization. PSUR collects the details related to the safety concerns of an authorized product in set intervals.

11.3   PSUR

PSUR = Periodic Safety Update Report

The PSUR has got a new identity with a new name the 'Periodic Benefit Risk Evaluation Report' or 'PBRER', (pronounced pee-brer). However, companies are still referring to the new PBRER as the PSUR.

PSUR presents the worldwide safety experience of a medicinal product at defined times post-authorization in order to: 👉

Report all the relevant new safety information from appropriate sources

Relate these data to patient exposure

Summarize the market authorization status in different countries and any significant variations related to safety

Create periodically the opportunity for an overall safety reevaluation

Indicate whether changes should be made to product information in order to optimize the use of the product

Fig: PSUR

11.4   PBRER

A PBRER is intended to present a periodic, comprehensive, concise and critical analysis of new or emerging information on the risks of the health product, and on its benefits in approved indications, to enable an appraisal of the product's overall benefit-risk profile.

This new concept represents an evolution of the traditional Periodic Safety Update Report (PSUR) from an interval safety report to a cumulative benefit-risk report. The "new" PSUR will evaluate not just the safety aspects of the drug the way the old PSUR did, but it will now evaluate the benefits of the drug. The benefits and risks will be weighed in the document and a benefit/risk (BR) evaluation will be made. It has changed the focus from individual case safety reports to aggregate data evaluation. In addition, the broadened scope of PBRER increased the need for integrating information within the report.

The PBRER retains most of the basic elements of the PSUR. Compared to the PSUR, the PBRER has more information on: 👉

Clinical trials and observational studies

Signals that are new, ongoing, or closed

Risk evaluation: signals (new, ongoing or closed), evaluation of risks and new information, and effectiveness of risk minimization activities.

Benefit evaluation: important baseline efficacy/effectiveness, evaluation of efficacy/effectiveness and new information.

Integrated risk-benefit analysis.

Fig: PBRER

So, PBRER is an important ingredient in a mission of protecting public health through its updated information regarding ongoing safety issues and emerging safety issue and detailed complex analysis of benefits, signals and risks (both known possible and unknown) associated with the drug.

To present a comprehensive picture of clinical safety, a medicinal product is required to be closely monitored throughout its lifecycle, especially during the first year of commercialization. Surveillance of marketed product is a shared responsibility of Marketing Authorization Holder (MAH) and Regulatory Authority. It is expected to provide concise summary information together with a critical evaluation of the risk-benefit balance of the product in the light of new or changing information.

11.5   Benefits of PBRER

Benefits of PBRER
Provides an opportunity for MAH to review the safety profile of their products and ensure that the product informations (e.g. SPC, PILs i.e. patient information leaflets) are up to date.
Helps Competent Authorities to monitor medicinal products by providing pharmacovigilance data.
Helps with critical risk - benefit evaluation of the product.

Fig: Benefits of PBRER

11.6   General Principles

11.7   Single PBRER for an Active Substance

- The PBRER should provide information on all approved indications, dosage forms, and regimens for the active substance, with a single data lock point. In some circumstances it will be appropriate to present data by indication, dosage form, dosing regimen, or population (e.g., children vs. adults) within the relevant section(s) of the PBRER. In exceptional cases, submission of separate PBRERs might be appropriate, for example an active substance used in two formulations for systemic and topical administration in entirely different indications.

- Safety information for the fixed combination may be reported either in a separate PBRER or included as separate presentations in the report for one of the separate components, depending on the circumstances.

- Cross referencing all relevant PBRER is considered important.

11.8 Products manufactured and/or marketed by more than one company

- Each MAH is responsible for submitting PBRER, even if different companies market the same product in the same country.

- When companies are involved in contractual relationships (e.g. licensor-licensee), arrangements for sharing safety information should be clearly specified.

11.9 Reference Information

- Reference information is required to compare that reported information in PBRER is in accord with previous knowledge on the drug's safety, and to indicate whether changes should be made to product information.

- CCSI (present in CCDS) is the reference information by which the listed and unlisted events are determined for the purpose of periodic reporting for marketed products, but it is not used for assessing the expectedness for expedited reporting.

Note: "Company Core Data Sheet" (CCDS) prepared by MAH includes information relating to safety, indications, dosing, pharmacology, and other information concerning the product.

11.10 Level of Detail within PBRER

- The level of detail provided in certain sections of the PBRER should depend on the medicinal product's known or emerging important benefits and risks.

  - For example, when there is important new safety information, a detailed presentation of that information and other relevant information (e.g., updated full benefit information) should be included to facilitate a robust benefit-risk analysis.

11.11 Benefit - Risk evaluation

- When a drug is approved for marketing, a conclusion has been reached that when the drug is used in accordance with approved product information, its benefits outweigh its risks.

- When a new information emerges about a marketed medicinal product, benefit-risk evaluation should be carried out to determine whether benefits continue to outweigh risks, and to consider whether steps need to be taken to improve the benefit-risk balance through risk minimization activities, e.g., labeling changes, communications with prescribers, or other steps.

11.12   Periodicity and PBRER data lock point

- Each medicinal product should have an International Birth Date (IBD), the date of the first marketing authorization for the product granted to any company in any country in the world. If desired by the MAH, the IBD can be designated as the last day of the same month.

- When a report contains information on different dosage forms, formulations, or uses (indications, routes, and populations), the date of the first marketing authorization for any of the various authorizations should be regarded as the IBD and, therefore, determines the data lock point for purposes of the PBRER.

- The data lock point is the date designated as the cutoff for data to be included in a PBRER.

- The need for a report and the frequency of report submission to authorities are subject to local regulatory requirements.

- As a result of the expanded scope of the PBRER, the time interval between the DLP and submission of PBRERs should be as follows:

    - PBRERs covering intervals of 6 or 12 months: within 70 calendar days
    - PBRERs covering intervals in excess of 12 months: within 90 calendar days
    - Ad hoc PBRERs: 90 calendar days, unless otherwise specified in the ad hoc request

The day of DLP is day 0 of the 70- or 90-calendar day interval between the DLP and report submission. Where national or regional requirements differ from the above, the MAH should discuss the timeline for submission with the relevant regulatory authority.

PBRER submissions are not required for all medicinal products, but the need for PBRER is determined using a risk-based approach. Certain products authorized under certain legal basis are exempted to submit PBRER routinely (generic, well-established, homeopathic and traditional herbal medicinal products). For such products, PBRER shall be submitted only where there is a condition in the marketing authorization or when requested by a competent authority. The PBRER submission frequency is variable.

11.13   Timelines - PBRER/PSUR

INDIA	US	EU	JAPAN
First 2 years: every 6 months	First 3 years: every 3 months	First 2 years: every 6 months	First 2 years: every 6 months
Next 2 years: annually	Annually thereafter	Next 2 years: annually	Annually thereafter
		3 yearly thereafter	

The PBRER is a more comprehensive document. The construction is modular so that sections can be used as is for other regulatory submissions e.g. risk management plan.
PBRER/PSUR can be an important pharmacovigilance tool by providing support:

- the identification of new safety signals

- a means of determining changes in the benefit-risk profile

- an effective means of risk communication to regulatory authorities

- an indicator for the need for risk management initiatives, as well as a tracking mechanism monitoring the effectiveness of such initiatives.

11.14   HBD - EU Harmonized Birth Date for submission of PBRER/PSUR

HBD – EU Harmonized Birth Date for submission of PBRER/PSUR

The International birth date (IBD) is the date of the first marketing authorization; the EU birth date is the date of the first authorization in Europe. Submission of PSUR/PBRER is normally determined by the date of national authorization which may differ in the various Member States. Thus, the same product of one marketing authorization holder can follow different PSUR /PBRER schemes in the various EU Member States. This results in duplicate work of both MAHs and competent authorities, which may even have negative impact on quality of the reports. Besides that, original medicinal products and generics usually have different birth dates and therefore it is difficult to ensure the same safety information in SPCs of similar products. The problems may be substantially reduced if all medicinal products with the same active substance have the same birth date within the EU, i.e. EU HBD (Harmonized birth date).

11.15 DSUR (Development Safety Update Report)

> **DSUR (Development Safety Update Report)**
>
> DSUR are safety document which covers safety profile of medicinal product during clinical trial and communicate to the Regulators and Ethics Committee at regular interval about adequate monitoring and evaluation of drug's safety profile. Sponsors are required to submit a DSUR within one year of the development International Birth Date (DIBD – the date of first authorization of a clinical trial in any country worldwide) and provide annual safety report until all open clinical studies have ended (clinical study is completed and study report has been submitted.) once the drug is authorized DSUR and PSUR/PBRER should be synchronized. Investigator brochure is used as the Reference Safety Information and SmPC is RSI for non commercial sponsors conducting trial with marketed product.

Twelve

SHORT NOTES

12.1 Introduction

This chapter contains brief notes on various topics which may help the reader to get further insight in to the subject of Pharmacovigilance. These notes are short, concise and clear thus making it easy for the reader to quickly recapitulate the concepts.

12.2 Narrative Writing

Individual Case Safety Reports (ICSRs) are vital drug safety documents required by health authorities for each medicinal product. Regulatory authorities mandate to write a narrative for all ICSRs for submission. Also, narratives give a stand-alone comprehensive and complete medical description of the case. So it is essential to ensure quality of the narrative.

A narrative is a detailed chronological description of the patient's adverse event experience. The objective of narrative writing is to summarize all relevant clinical and related information, including:

- Patient characteristics

- Diagnosis

- Therapy Details

- Medical History

- Narrative of Clinical events

- Known adverse reactions alongside the relevant outcome

- Results of laboratory tests along with the normal ranges

- Any other information that refutes or confirms an adverse reaction

The information should be presented in a logical time sequence; ideally this should be presented in the chronology of patient's experience, rather than in the chronology in which the information was received.

These narratives summarize the details surrounding the event to enable understanding of the circumstances that may have led to the occurrence of the AE and its subsequent management.

Basic rules for narrative writing

- Correct use of grammar

- Medical content (relevant)

- Chronology

- Writing in past/third tense

As well as inclusion of component items, the report must follow the formatting guideline as a matter of obligation rather than the regulators preference.

Various sources of information for narratives:

- CIOMS Forms (Council for International Organizations of Medical Sciences forms)

- CRFs (Case Report Forms)

- MedWatch Forms

- DCFs (Data Clarification Forms)

- Clinical Database listings

Narrative formation process

The narrative formation process varies company to company. Although template of narrative varies (flexible) according to sponsor's/company's requirements but the internal consistency should be maintained to include all relevant information in relevant sequence to give a complete guide to AE occurrence and its management. A generalized template is discussed here:

Identifying information

The information in the top identifies Reporter, Report type (Spontaneous report/study report) and Dayo.

The Body of the Narrative

Body of narrative should provide enough information to medical reviewer to understand (what happened/ why happened/when happened) clearly the complete picture of adverse event.

The first paragraph:

- Patient details, suspect drug(s), indication (known/unknown).

- Medical history/social history and concomitant medications

The second paragraph:

- Description of event (chronological order) i.e.

    - Intake of drug

    - Occurrence of event

    - Action taken with the drug

    - Outcome of event

The final paragraph:

Causality detail is given by reporter between reported adverse event and suspected drug.

12.3 ICH - (International Conference on Harmonization of Technical Requirements for Registration of Pharmaceuticals for Human Use)

Establishment of ICH - April 1990, in Brussels.
ICH is unique in bringing together the regulatory authorities and pharmaceutical industry of Europe, Japan and the US to discuss scientific and technical aspects of drug registration.

Objective of ICH

To increase international harmonization of technical requirements to ensure that safe, effective, and high quality medicines are developed and registered in the most efficient and cost-effective manner in order to:

- To promote public health

- Prevent unnecessary duplication of clinical trials in humans

- Minimize the use of animal testing without compromising safety and effectiveness.

Goal of ICH

- Promote international harmonization by bringing together representatives from the three ICH regions (EU, Japan and USA) to discuss and establish common guidelines.

- Promote mutual understanding regarding regional initiatives to maintain harmonization related to ICH guidelines regionally and globally and to strengthen the capacity of drug regulatory authorities and industry to utilize them.

- Provide information on request by any company/country regarding guidelines/activities of ICH.

Members of ICH

- ICH is comprised of representatives from six parties that represent the regulatory bodies and research-based industry in the European Union, Japan and the USA.

- In Japan, the members are the Ministry of Health, Labour and Welfare (MHLW), and the Japan Pharmaceutical Manufacturers Association (JPMA).

- In Europe, the members are the European Union (EU), and the European Federation of Pharmaceutical Industries and Associations (EFPIA).

- In Europe, the members are the European Union (EU), and the European Federation of Pharmaceutical Industries and Associations (EFPIA).

- In the USA, the members are the Food and Drug Administration (FDA), and the Pharmaceutical Research and Manufacturers of America (PhRMA).

- Additional members include Observers from the World Health Organization (WHO) European Free Trade Association (EFTA, currently represented by Swissmedic), and Canada (Health Canada).

- The International Federation of Pharmaceutical Manufacturers & Associations (IFPMA) has been closely involved with ICH since its inception.

ICH Location

No office for ICH because it is a voluntary cooperative effort of cosponsors from the three regions. The ICH Secretariat is based in Geneva. The biannual meetings and conferences of the ICH Steering Committee rotate between the EU, Japan, and the USA.

12.4   WHO (World Health Organization)

WHO is specialized agency of the United Nations (UN) that is concerned with international public health.
Establishment of WHO - 7 April 1948, headquartered in Geneva, Switzerland.

WHO responsibilities:

- Providing leadership on global health matters

- Shaping the health research agenda ,stimulating the generation, translation and dissemination of valuable knowledge

- Setting norms and standards, promoting and monitoring their implementation

- Articulating ethical and evidence-based policy options

- Providing technical support, catalyzing change, and building sustainable institutional capacity

- Monitoring the health situation and assessing health trends

12.5   UMC (Uppsala Monitoring Centre)

UMC is World Health Organization Collaborating Centre and responsible for management of WHO programme for International Drug Monitoring.
Establishment of UMC - 1978,located in Uppsala, Sweden

The work of the UMC is:

- To co-ordinate the WHO Programme for International Drug Monitoring and its more than 100 member countries

- To collect, assess and communicate information from member countries about the benefits, harms and risks of drugs and other substances used in medicine to improve patient therapy and public health worldwide

- To collaborate with member countries in the development and practice of the science of pharmacovigilance

12.6   Vigibase, VigiFlow, Vigimed, VigiSearch, VigiMine

VigiBase

VigiBase is the name of the WHO global ICSR database.   It is a unique collection of international drug safety data.
It consists of reports of adverse reactions received from member countries since 1968.
The VigiBase data resource is the largest and most comprehensive in the world.
It is developed and maintained by the UMC on behalf of the World Health Organization.
VigiBase is a computerized pharmacovigilance system, in which information is recorded in a structured, hierarchical form to allow for easy and flexible retrieval and analysis of the data.
Its purpose is to provide the evidence from which potential medicine safety hazards may be detected.

VigiFlow

VigiFlow is a complete ICSR management system created and maintained by the UMC. It is web-based and built to adhere to the ICH-E2B standard. It can be used as the national database for countries in the WHO Programme as it incorporates tools for report analysis, and facilitate sending reports to VigiBase.

Vigimed

Vigimed share point based conferencing facility, exclusive to member countries of the WHO Programme for International Drug Monitoring for fast communication of topical pharmacovigilance issues.

VigiSearch

VigiSearch is a search service for accessing ICSRs stored in the VigiBase database offered by the UMC to national pharmacovigilance centres and other third- party inquirers.

VigiMine

VigiMine - a statistical tool within VigiSearch with vast statistical material calculated for all Drug-ADR pairs (combinations) available in VigiBase. The main features include the disproportionality measure (IC value) stratified in different ways and useful filter capabilities.

12.7 EudraVigilance

(European Union Drug Regulating Authorities Pharmaco**vigilance**)
EudraVigilance is a system designed for the reporting of suspected adverse effects.
It is the European data processing network and management system for reporting and evaluation of suspected adverse reactions during the development of new drugs and for following the marketing authorization of medicinal products in the European Economic Area (EEA).
The European Medicines Agency is responsible for the development, maintenance and coordination of EudraVigilance.
The European EudraVigilance system deals with :

- Electronic exchange of Individual Case Safety Reports

- Early detection of possible safety signals from marketed drugs for human use.

- Continuous monitoring and evaluation of potential safety issues in relation to reported adverse reactions.

- Decision making process, based on a broader knowledge of the adverse reaction profile of drugs.

EudraVigilance facilitates the process of risk management at several levels including aspects of risk detection, risk assessment, risk minimization and risk communication.
In short, EudraVigilance contributes to:

- Protection and promotion of public health in the EEA

- Provides a powerful tool for monitoring the safety of medicinal products

- Minimizing potential risks related to suspected adverse reactions

12.8 QPPV (Qualified Person Responsible for Pharmacovigilance)

A QPPV is an individual of a company who ensures that MAH (Marketing Authorization Holder) meets its legal obligations for the monitoring of the safety of the product within the EU market.
Anyone marketing a medicinal product in any of the Member States of the European Union (EU) or the 3 EEA Member States (Iceland, Liechtenstein and Norway) must have a QPPV.
The QPPV has to live within the EU/EEA, being accessible on a 24/7 basis and has to have a back up (Deputy QPPV).
The PSMF (Pharmacovigilance System Master File) must be accessible to the QPPV at any time.

Responsibilities of QPPV:

- Ensures MAH has an appropriate Pharmacovigilance system in place

- MAH have an overview of safety profile of their products

- To be a point of contact with the competent authorities

- Responsible for reports like ICSR/PSUR to Competent authorities

Required criteria for appointing QPPV:

- Appropriately qualified(medically qualified/has access to a medically qualified person)

- Knowledge and experience in working in Pharmacovigilance

- Documented experience in all aspects of Pharmacovigilance

12.9   PV Metrics

It is difficult to manage without measures .PV metrics assess performance and improvement of PV system.

Key Performance Indicators in Pharmacovigilance:

- Time Metrics (time needed to complete a work)

- Quality Metrics (quality of work done)

- Productivity Metrics (work done per day/month by an associate)

Time Metrics can be defined by case type, time taken for reviewing (Quality check) a case percentage of cases reported within 15 days from receipt.

Quality metrics can be defined by number and type of errors. For example, number of error per case.

Productivity Metrics can be defined by total number of case handled/per associate/per day/per role and total number of reported working days for each associate.

These three metrics helps to determine the success of an individual as well as success of company. Metrics lead to better decisions and better spending as it helps to:

- Tracks progress and performance

- Evaluates impact

- Improves accountability

12.10   Inspection and Audit and Monitoring

Inspection

The act by a regulatory authority(ies) of conducting an official review of documents, facilities, records, and any other resources that are deemed by the authority(ies) to be related to the clinical trial and that may be located at the site of the trial, at the sponsor's and/or contract research organizations (CROs) facilities, or at other establishments deemed appropriate by the regulatory authority (ies).

Audit

A systematic and independent examination of trial-related activities and documents to determine whether the evaluated trial-related activities were conducted, and the data were recorded, analyzed, and accurately reported according to the protocol, sponsor's standard operating procedures (SOPs), good clinical practice (GCP), and the applicable regulatory requirement(s).

In simple words, Audit is the systematic examination (verification) of a Process/System/Procedure.

Audit can be :

- Routine Audit (to ensure processes are compliant) and

- For-cause Audit (when there is doubt/evidence that process is non-compliant)

Inspection and Audit are same but when audit is done by Regulatory Authority (& more serious) it is called inspection.

Reasons for Audit/Inspection

In a clinical study if there are

- Any concerns about its safety, data or ethics

- Requirement of monitoring standards of clinical research

- Suspicion of fraud/scientific misconduct

- Serious quality systems breakdown

Differences between Inspection and Audit

Inspection	Audit
Inspectors are employed by government, through the agency of regulatory body.(such appointed by FDA)	Inspectors/Auditors are employed by the Sponsor or independent consultant can also perform this task.
To ensure that a site is complying with protocol, SOP, GCP and Applicable regulatory requirements.	To ensure trial related obligations and acceptability of resultant clinical data is in support of a new drug approval.

Monitoring

The act of overseeing the progress of a clinical trial, and of ensuring that it is conducted recorded, and reported in accordance with the protocol, standard operating procedures (SOPs) GCP, and the applicable regulatory requirement(s).

Monitoring is a quality control continuous process during entire clinical trial, generall performed by CRA.

12.11   Schedule Y

Schedule Y is the requirements and guidelines for permission to import and / or manufactur of new drugs for sale or to undertake clinical trials in India.

In short: It is the law that drives Clinical Trials in India.

12.12   HIPAA (Health Insurance portability and Accountability Act)

It is a "Privacy Rule" implemented by Federal Government.

The Privacy Rule standards address :

- The use and disclosure of individuals' health information called "protected healt information(PHI)" by organizations subject to the Privacy Rule - called "covere entities,"

- Individuals' privacy rights to understand and control how their health information used.

PHI - is the information that identifies an individual and relates to the person's physical/ment health or condition, the provision of healthcare to that person or payment for the provision c healthcare to that person.

PHI includes: patient's names, addresses and all other information pertaining to the patient health and payment records.

HIPPA protects individual's rights to control access to and disclosure of private and confidential information.

Difference between "USE" and "DISCLOSURE"

USE - Within organization /under direct control of organization.
Example: CRC (Clinical research coordinator) uses study subject PHI when observing subject.

DISCLOSURE - PHI given to a person who is not the part of organization.
Example : CRA (Clinical research associate) looks into the study subject source documents

12.13   Ethics Committee

Ethics committee can be classified as Independent committee (IRB/IEC) and Central Ethics Committee (CEC).

Need for Ethics Committee

- To protect human subjects To check for ethical values i.e.

    – Beneficence (Do good)

    – Non-Maleficence (Do not harm)

    – Autonomy ((Respect for the person)

    – Justice

    – Dignity(confidentiality)

    – Truthfulness & Honesty (informed consent)

    – No influence /coercion justice

The responsibility of an ethics committee is to ensure the protection of the rights, safety and well-being of participants involved in clinical research.

Where Does Ethics Committee work?

Prior the trial begins :
- Review the trial
- Decide upon the trial

During the trial :
- Continue reviewing
- Check/monitor for adverse events

End of the trial :
- Review of report
- Record keeping

IRB/IEC

An institutional review board (IRB), also known as an independent ethics committee (IEC), ethical review board (ERB) or research ethics board (REB), is a committee that has been formally designated to approve, monitor, and review biomedical and behavioral research involving humans.

Differences between IRB and IEC

IRB	IEC
Members of IRB are attached Institutions/ Organization	Members of IEC are independent or more than one organization .
Review project of the Institutions	Review project of all the applicant
Meetings are in the institution premises	Meeting venue is decide by members
Usually termed in U.S. and other countries	Usually called in India

12.14   GCP (Good Clinical Practice)

GCP is defined as a standard for the design, conduct, performance, monitoring, auditing, recording, analyses and reporting of clinical trials.
Compliance with GCP ensures:

 • Data and reported results during trial are credible and accurate and

 • Rights, integrity and confidentiality of trial subjects are protected

GCP:

 • Are mainly focused on the protection of human rights in clinical trial.

 • Provide assurance of the safety of the newly developed compounds.

 • Provide standards on how clinical trials should be conducted.

- Define the roles and responsibilities of clinical sponsors, clinical research investigators, Clinical Research Associates, and monitors.

GCPs are generally accepted, international best practices for conducting clinical trials and device studies.

GCP are made up of:

- FDA regulations and guidance document

- ICH guidelines

- Codes of ethical conduct (Declaration of Helsinki and The Nuremburg Code)

The Nuremburg Code of 1947 The Nuremberg Code is a set of research ethics principles for human experimentation set as a result of the Subsequent Nuremberg Trials at the end of the Second World War.

Declaration of Helsinki In 1964, the World Medical Association established recommendations guiding medical doctors in biomedical research involving human subjects.

12.15   Difference between Patient Safety Report and ICSR (Individual Case Safety Report)

Patient Safety Report	ICSR(Individual Case Safety Report)
Describes all relevant events for a single patient with relevant background information	Describes one patient, one or more identifiable reporter, one or more suspected adverse reaction(s) that are clinically and temporarily associated and one or more suspected medicinal product(s)
Related to Clinical Study report(CSR)	Related to PV services/drug safety

12.16   Clinical Research

Research is a systematic investigation to establish fact. Treatment is the care provided to improve a situation.

Clinical research is a systematic observational and experimental biomedical study performed in human subject to study drug/device/biologics/surgery/radiotherapy for its safe and therapeutic use.

Ultimate goal of Clinical Research is to improve quality of life.

Importance of Research:

- New drugs to market

- New methods for surgery

- New combination of standard therapy

- New approach for radiation therapy

- New techniques for screening and diagnosing a disease

- New techniques such as gene therapy

Research Impact:

- Build the scientific foundation for clinical practice

- Prevent disease and disability

- Manage and eliminate symptoms caused by illness

- Enhance end-of-life care (end-of-life care refers to healthcare, not only of patients in th final hours/days of their lives, but more broadly care of all those with a terminal illness o terminal condition that has become advanced, progressive and incurable.) and palliativ care (Palliative care is medical care that relieves pain/ symptoms/ stress caused by seriou illnesses, improving patients' quality of life. e.g. Comfort care given to a patient sufferin; from cancer from the time of diagnosis and throughout the course of illness.

- Help in decision making process

Ethical norms in Clinical Research:

Three ethical principles guide clinical research

- Respect for person

- Beneficence- do no harm, or maximize possible benefits and minimize possible harm

- Justice - treatment of all fairly and all equally share benefits and risks

Clinical research includes:

- Medical and behavioral research involving volunteer participants
- Investigations that are carefully developed and conducted with clinical outcomes recorded
- Identification of better ways to prevent, diagnose, treat, and understand human disease
- Trials that test new treatments, clinical management and clinical outcomes, and long-term studies
- Strict scientific guidelines
- Ethical principles to protect participants

Examples of Clinical research types:

Clinical trials/therapeutic research - disease diagnosis and prognosis(prediction of the probable course and outcome of a disease), Clinical decision making
Clinical Economics - cost effectiveness of healthcare
Disease epidemiology - incidence, prevalence, distribution of risk factors for specific disease .

12.17   Line Listing and Summary Tabulation

Line Listing

A format of drug safety report required by regulatory authorities that provides key information but not necessarily all of the details customarily found in an ICSR.
It serves to help regulatory authorities identify cases they might wish to examine more completely by requesting full case report.

Summary Tabulation

Summary Tabulation is aggregate summary of each of Line Listing.
The requirement of Line Listing and Summary Tabulation depends on the type or source of adverse drug reaction.

12.18   Thalidomide Disaster

Thalidomide was used for sound sleep (sedative) especially in pregnant women having symptoms related to morning sickness.
At that time it was not realized by scientists that drug taken by a pregnant woman could pass across the placental barrier and harm the developing fetus. But, unfortunately it happened and

thousands of babies got affected which ended up with disabled babies and even death. Catastrophic results:

- Peripheral neuritis - nerve disorder

- Birth defects - deafness, blindness, disfigurement, cleft palate, internal defects phocomelia(bilateral shortened limbs-arms and legs)

Kefauver Harris Amendment (1962) was implemented in response to this tragedy.
It introduced a requirement for drug manufacturers to provide proof of the effectiveness and safety of their drugs before approval.

12.19   Sulfanilamide Tragedy

Sulfanilamide, a drug used to treat streptococcal infections, had been used safely for some time in tablet and powder form.
In June 1937, however, a salesman for the S.E. Massengill Co., in Bristol, reported a demand in the southern states for the drug in liquid form.
Liquid form of Sulfanilamide produced using diethylene glycol as solvent.
Existing laws did not require any kind of pharmacological studies demonstrating that a drug is safe.
Diethylene glycol = Antifreeze
Because no pharmacological studies had been done on the new sulfanilamide preparation Watkins failed to note one characteristic of the solution. Diethylene glycol, a chemical normally used as antifreeze, is a deadly poison.
It caused the deaths of more than 100 people.
This tragedy prompted passage of Federal Food, Drug, and Cosmetic Act (1938).

12.20   Pharmacoepidemiology

Pharmacoepidemiology is the study of the uses and effects of drugs in well defined populations
It provides an estimate of the probability of beneficial effects of a drug in a population and the probability of adverse effects.
Pharmacoepidemiology has become one of the important contributors in understanding drug safety issues. One good example is confirmation and quantification of the relation between NSAID treatment and gastrointestinal ulceration and bleeding.
Pharmacoepidemiology is a bridge between clinical pharmacology and epidemiology. (Clinical pharmacology is the study of effect of drugs on clinical humans and Epidemiology is the study of the distribution and determinants of diseases and other health states in populations.)
Pharmacovigilance is a part of pharmacoepidemiology that involves continual monitoring of

safety concern and adverse effects related to a medicinal product.

Pharmacoepidemiology sometimes also involves the conduct and evaluation of programmatic efforts to improve medication use on a population basis.

Pharmacoepidemiological studies are largely based on observational rather than experimental data.

12.21   Patent

Patent is a Copyright.

A government authority or license conferring a right or title for a set period, especially the sole right to exclude others from making, using, or selling an invention.

In simple words, patent is a legal protection which gives an innovator sole right to make, use and sell their invention for a set period of time.

In the field of pharmaceutical inventions, a product patent gives protection to a chemical/biological compound (The active component of a medicine), also called a "New Chemical Entity" (NCE) or Active Pharmaceutical Ingredient (API).

Legal term of a patent is normally 20 years from filing the "effective patent term", defined as the length of time in which a product (pharmaceutical and agrochemical products) is marketed with the benefit of enforceable patent protection.

12.22   Brand Name Drug and Generic Drug

Brand Name Drug

A brand name drug is a drug marketed under a proprietary, trademark-protected name.

A brand name drug is a drug that has a trade name and is protected by a patent (legal protection that gives innovator company sole right to make, use and sell their invention for set period of time). Company produces brand name drug is known as "Innovator company" as they invent the drug.

It takes 10-15 years and a high cost (over $1billion)for a brand name drug which passes through several research and testing in animals and humans to be available for general public. During this testing, the company making the drug must prove that it is safe and effective for people to use. Once the new drug is approved, the company that made and tested it receives a patent which provides legal protection to the drug i.e. no one can copy the drug till patent is valid which takes around 20 years to expire.

Generic Drug

A medicine with the same active ingredient, but not necessarily the same inactive ingredients as a brand-name drug. A generic drug may be marketed only after the original drug's patent has expired.

A generic drug is a copy of a brand name drug. To get permission from Regulatory Authority for marketing generic product, manufacturers (generic companies) must prove that their generic drug is "bioidentical" i.e. same as the original brand name drug in the following ways:

- Dosage form (tablet, capsule, liquid, etc.)

- Strength (same amount of drug in both)

- Safety and quality

- How it is taken (by mouth, injection, etc.)

- How the medicine gets into the bloodstream and works in the body

Once the patent for a drug under a specific brand expires, any other company can copy the drug and sell a generic version of that drug. To produce a generic drug, the generic company has to prove only that their product is the same as the product of the specific brand for which the generic company does not need to spend much time and money because they do not need to go through all processes like brand name drug goes through. They do BABE studies for proving their product is bioidentical to brand name drug.

An example of a generic drug, one used for diabetes, is metformin. A brand name for metformin is Glucophage. (Brand names are usually capitalized while generic names are not.) A generic drug, one used for hypertension, is metoprolol, whereas a brand name for the same drug is Lopressor.

12.23   Black Triangle Drug

When new drugs and vaccines are first marketed they are intensively monitored in order to confirm the risk/benefit profile of the product. Such products are labeled with an inverted black triangle ▼.

Healthcare professionals are encouraged to report all suspected ADRs which occur as a result of the use of all black triangle drugs regardless of the seriousness of the reaction.

Newly marketed drugs will usually be intensively monitored for a minimum of two years.

It should be noted, however, that a black triangle is not always removed after this length of time and any medication can be assigned a black triangle if it is considered that it needs to be intensively monitored.

For example, black triangle status may be re-assigned to an established product if it is granted a new indication or route of administration, if it is marketed as a new combination with another established active ingredient, or if it is targeted towards a new patient population. .

12.24   Overdose, Medication error, Drug misuse and Drug Abuse

Overdose

A drug overdose is the accidental or intentional use of a drug or medicine in an amount that is higher than is normally used.

Medication Error

Any incorrect or wrongful administration of a medication, such as incorrect dosage, drug, patient, time or route of administration, interaction between incompatible medications, failure to prescribe or administer the correct drug for a particular disease/ condition, use of outdated drugs.

Drug Misuse

When a person takes a legal prescription medication for a purpose other than the reason it was prescribed, or when that person takes a drug not prescribed to him or her, that is misuse of a drug. Misuse can include taking a drug in a manner or at a dose that was not recommended by a health care professional. This can happen when the person hopes to get a bigger or faster therapeutic response from medications such as sleeping or weight loss pills.

In other words, inappropriate use of prescribed or non- prescribed medicine, but not for "pleasure" or other non-medicinal purposes.

Examples :

A common example is "more will work better." For instance, if a person isn't able to fall asleep after taking a single sleeping pill, he may take another pill an hour later, thinking, "That will do the job."

Another examples of drug misuse are;

A person may offer his headache medication to a friend who is in pain.

Another is to stop taking an antibiotic before the pills have been completely taken.

These are drug misuse where people are not looking to "get high" but they are also not following medical instructions.

Drug Abuse

Misusing a drug to such an extent that it becomes addiction and willful habit or we can sa repeatedly and willfully using a drug in a way other than prescribed or socially sanctioned. It i mostly related to individual's intentions or motivations.

For example, a person knows that he will get a pleasant or euphoric feeling by taking the drug especially at higher doses than prescribed. That is an example of drug abuse because the perso is specifically looking for that euphoric response.

12.25   Drug addiction and Drug Dependence

Drug addiction

Drug addiction can be defined as a condition characterized by an overwhelming desire t continue taking a drug to which one has become habituated through repeated consumptio because it produces a particular effect, usually an alteration of mental status.

Addiction is usually accompanied by

- A compulsion to obtain the drug

- A tendency to increase the dose

- A psychologic or physical dependence

- Detrimental consequences for the individual and society

Common addictive drugs are barbiturates, alcohol, morphine and other opioids, especiall heroin, which has slightly greater euphorigenic properties than other opium.

Drug Dependence

Drug dependence means that a person needs a drug to function normally.
Dependence is usually accompanied by

- Abruptly stopping the drug leads to withdrawal symptoms.

- No strong motivation to continue the use of these substances.

- A person may have a physical dependence on a substance without having an addiction.

For example, certain blood pressure medications do not cause addiction but they can caus physical dependence.

In a nutshell, Drug Dependence and Drug Addiction are distinct from each other. Afte taking a drug for a long time, someone might increase their tolerance to it and have unpleasan withdrawal symptoms if they quit using, this is called physical dependence whereas if someone is using drugs for the wrong reasons and also allows them mess up his/her life but continues using them in spite of that knowledge, he/she is addicted.

12.26   Clinical trial in a nutshell

CLINICAL TRIAL: Clinical trials, also known as clinical studies, test potential treatments (drug, medical device, or biologic, such as a vaccine, blood product, or gene therapy) in human volunteers or patients to see whether they should be further investigated or approved for wider use in the general population.

Potential treatments, however, must first be studied in laboratory models or animals to determine its safety before they can be tried in people. Treatments having acceptable safety profiles for the disease or condition and showing the most promise are then moved into clinical trials. Clinical trials are an integral part of new product discovery and development, and are required by all regulatory agencies (e.g., the Food and Drug Administration (FDA) in the United States), before a new product can be brought to the market.

Generalized process flow of clinical trial is mentioned below:

- Protocol is approved for clinical study/trial.

- Investigator and co-workers are selected for conducting trial related activities.

- Approval is taken for the processes involved in the trial.

- Patient recruitment process is completed and participation of patient in the trial is started.

- Data entry is done for the information collected during clinical trial process.

- Statistical Analysis of collected data is completed.

- Presentation and publication of analyzed report is done.

- Completed reports of clinical trial filed and registration is obtained from Regulatory Authority

Definitions related to clinical trial

Clinical Trial

Any investigation in human subjects intended to determine the clinical pharmacological, pharmacokinetic, and/or other pharmacodynamic effects of an investigational product, and/or to identify any adverse reactions to an investigational product to assess the product's safety and efficacy.

Protocol

Protocol is a written plan for carrying out a clinical study. A protocol includes what will be done, when, and how.

Or,

A protocol is the study plan on which a clinical trial is based. Each trial is carefully designed to safeguard the health of participants as well as answer specific research questions. A protocol describes what types of people may participate in the trial, the schedule of tests, procedures, medications, dosages, and length of the study.

Standard Operating Procedure (SOP)

Official, detailed, written instructions for the management of clinical trials. SOPs ensure that all the functions and activities of a clinical trial are carried out in a consistent and efficient manner.

Investigator's Brochure

Relevant clinical and non-clinical data compiled on the investigational drug, biologic or device being studied.

Ethics Committee

An independent group of both medical and non-medical professionals who are responsible for verifying the integrity of a study and ensuring the safety, integrity, and human rights of the study participants.

Compliance (In Relation to Clinical Trials)

Adherence to all the trial-related requirements, good clinical practice (GCP), ethical requirements, and the applicable regulatory requirements.

Applicable regulatory requirement

Any law(s) and regulation(s) addressing the conduct of clinical trials of investigational products of the jurisdiction where trial is conducted.

Case Report Form (CRF)

A record of pertinent information collected on each subject during a clinical trial, as outlined in the study protocol.

Sponsor

An individual, company, institution or organization which takes responsibility for the initiation, management, and / or financing of a clinical trial.

The sponsor does not actually conduct the investigation unless the sponsor is a sponsor-investigator.

CRO (Contract Research Organization)

A person or an organization (commercial, academic or other) contracted by the sponsor to perform one or more of a sponsor's study-related duties and functions.

Or,

A contract research organization (CRO) is an organization that provides support to the pharmaceutical, biotechnology, and medical device industries in the form of research services outsourced on a contract basis.

Investigator

A medical professional, usually a physician but may also be a nurse, pharmacist or other health care professional, under whose direction an investigational drug is administered or dispensed.

Principal Investigator

A person responsible for the overall conduct of the clinical trial at a trial site. If a trial is conducted by a team of individuals at a trial site, the investigator is the responsible leader of the team and may be called the principal investigator.

Coordinating Investigator

An investigator assigned the responsibility for the coordination of investigators at different centers participating in a multicenter trial.

CRA(Clinical Research Associate) or Monitor

Person who visits the site periodically during trial to monitor the data and assesses the progress of trial.

or,

Person employed by the study sponsor or CRO to monitor clinical study at all participating sites and reviews study records to determine that a study is being conducted in accordance with the protocol.

Clinical Research Coordinator (CRC)

Person at clinical trial site who manages daily operations of clinical trial at site and responsible to investigator.

Human Subject

A patient or healthy individual participating in a research study voluntarily.

Source Documentation

Location where information is first recorded including original documents, data and records.

Source Data

All information contained in original records and certified copies of results, observations or other facets required for the reconstruction and evaluation of the study that is contained in source documents.

Blinding

The process through which one or more parties to a clinical trial are unaware of the treatment assignments. In a single-blinded study, usually the subjects are unaware of the treatment assignments. In a double-blinded study, both the subjects and the investigators are unaware of the treatment assignments. Also, in a double-blinded study, the monitors and sometimes the data analysts are unaware. "Blinded" studies are conducted to prevent the unintentional biases that can affect subject data when treatment assignments are known.

Open-Label Trial

A clinical trial in which doctors and participants know which treatment is being administered.

Randomization

A process of assigning treatment to subject by using an element of "by chance" to reduce bias.

Bias

When a point of view prevents impartial judgment on issues relating to the subject of that point of view. In clinical studies, bias is controlled by blinding and randomization.

Informed Consent process

A process by which a subject voluntarily confirms his/her willingness to participate in a particular trial after having been informed about all aspects of clinical trial which are relevant to subject's participation decision.

Informed Consent Document

A document explaining all relevant study information to assist the study volunteer in understanding the expectations and requirements of participation in a clinical trial. This document is presented to and signed by the study subject.
Or,
A document that describes the rights of the study participants, and includes details about the study, such as its purpose, duration, required procedures, and key contacts. Risks and potential benefits are explained in the informed consent document. The participant will be asked to sign this document if they agree to participate in the trial. The informed consent document is not a contract. Participation in the clinical trial is voluntary and the participant may withdraw from the trial at any time without penalty or loss of benefits to which he/she is otherwise entitled.

Assent

A child's consent to participate in a clinical trial.

Confidentiality

The assurance that a participant's information will be kept secret and that access to that information is limited to authorized persons.

Enrolling

The act of signing up participants into a study. Generally this process involves evaluating a participant with respect to the eligibility criteria of the study and going through the informed consent process.

Eligibility Criteria

Summary criteria for participant selection; includes inclusion and exclusion criteria .

Exclusion /Inclusion criteria

There are characteristics that must be present (inclusion) or absent (exclusion) in order for a subject to qualify for a trial as per the protocol of the trial.

The medical or social standards determining whether a person may or may not be allowed to enter a clinical trial. These criteria are based on factors such as age, gender, pregnancy status, the type and stage of a disease, previous treatment history, and other medical conditions. It is important to note that inclusion and exclusion criteria are not used to reject people personally, but rather to identify appropriate participants to ensure the integrity of the study and to keep them safe.

Comparator Drug (Product)

An investigational or marketed product (i.e., active control) or placebo, used as a reference in clinical trial.

Experimental Drug (product)

A drug that is not FDA licensed for use in humans, or as a treatment for a particular condition.

Experimental group

The group of subjects exposed to the new, researched treatment. This group is often compared to a 'control group'(the subjects who are not exposed to that treatment).

Control Group

A comparison group of study subjects who are not treated with the investigational agent. The subjects in this group may receive no therapy, a different therapy, or a placebo.

Placebo

A placebo is an inactive pill, liquid, or powder that has no treatment value. In clinical trials, experimental treatments are often compared with placebos to assess the treatment's effectiveness.

Placebo Controlled Trial

A method of drug investigation in which an inactive substance (a placebo) is given to one group of participants, while the drug being tested is given to another group. The results obtained in the two groups are then compared to see if the investigational treatment is more effective than the placebo in treating the condition.

Placebo Effect

A physical or emotional change, occurring after an inactive substance is taken or administered that is not the result of any special property of the substance. The change may be beneficial reflecting the expectations of the participant and, often, the expectations of the person giving the substance.

Randomized Trial

A study in which participants are randomly (i.e., by chance) assigned to one of two or more treatment arms of a clinical trial.

Arm

Arm can be defined as any of the treatment groups in a clinical trial. Most randomized trials have two "arms," but some have three "arms," or even more.

Controlled Trials

A control is a standard against which experimental observations may be evaluated. In a controlled clinical trial, one group of participants is given an experimental drug, while another group (i.e., the control group) is given either a standard treatment for the disease or a placebo.

Crossover Trial

A clinical trial in which all participants receive both treatments, but at different times. At a predetermined point in the study, one group is switched from the experimental treatment to the control treatment (standard treatment), and the other group is switched from the control to the experimental treatment.

Parallel trial(study)

A parallel designed clinical trial compares the results of a treatment on two separate groups of patients. The sample size calculated for a parallel design can be used for any study where two groups are being compared.

Multicenter Trial

Clinical trial conducted according to a single protocol but at more than one site, and, therefore, carried out by more than one investigator.

Endpoint

Overall outcome that the protocol is designed to evaluate.

Clinical Study/Trial Report

A written description of a study of any therapeutic, prophylactic, or diagnostic agent conducted in human subjects, in which the clinical and statistical description, presentations, and analysi are fully integrated into a single report.

Biologic

A virus, therapeutic serum, toxin, antitoxin, vaccine, blood, blood component or derivative allergenic product, or analogous product applicable to the prevention, treatment or cure o diseases or injuries of human.

12.27   EU Regulation for Pharmaceutical Product Registration

National procedure

Each EU Member State has its own procedure for the authorisation of medicinal product tha fall outside the scope of the centralized procedure.

Applicants must submit an application to the competent authority of the Member State. Fo instance, in UK, MHRA is the competent authority.

"Competent authority is the competent official organization empowered to execute variou functions. Its responsibility may include the management of official systems of inspection o certification at the regional or local level."

Any pharmaceutical product which needs a marketing authorization in order to be sold in on or more EU countries needs to follow one of the following legal routes:

- Centralized Procedure (CP)

- Mutual Recognition Procedure (MRP)

- Decentralized Procedure(DCP)

When a medicinal product does not fall within the mandatory scopes of the CP,the applican may apply for marketing authorization in one or several countries in the European Union b using the Mutual Recognition Procedure (MRP) or the Decentralized Procedure (DCP), i which case the competent authorities of the Member States are responsible for granting th authorizations. At the end of a successful procedure, the medicinal product receives one o several national marketing authorizations in the selected countries. In both the MRP an the DCP, the applicant should request one Member State to act as Reference Member Stat (RMS). It is the RMS that prepares an Assessment Report on the medicinal product and send to the other Concerned Member State(s) (CMS/s) where the applicant would like marketin authorization in.

Centralized Procedure

Centralized procedure results in a single marketing authorisation that is valid in all EU countries, as well as in the European Economic Area (EEA) countries (Iceland, Liechtenstein and Norway). EMA is responsible for legal administration of marketing authorisation process.

A single application is made with the aim of gaining marketing authorisation throughout all the countries of the EU, Iceland, Norway and Liechtenstein.

Once a product is launched into the market, the European Commission is then the responsible agency for the product activity.

One of the EU countries regulatory authority becomes the official Rapporteur, and will be responsible for the initial assessments for the Marketing Authority application. A second agency is appointed as the official Co-Rapporteur who shares the responsibility for safety assessment and monitoring of the product, once product is launched into the market.

The Committee for Medicinal Products for Human Use (CHMP) is the committee at the European Medicines Agency that is responsible for preparing opinions on questions concerning medicines for human use.

Mutual Recognition Procedure

Mutual Recognition Procedure is required when a product possesses a marketing authorisation issued by a single EU country but is required to be marketed in other EU countries or it can be explained as companies that have a product authorized in one EU Member State can apply for this authorisation to be recognized in other EU countries through Mutual Recognition Procedure.

The nation which issued the marketing authorisation on a national level is known as the 'Reference Member State'.

The other countries where the product is applying to be sold in, are known as the 'Concerned Member States'.

If the application is successful, the marketing authorisation issued by reference Member State is copied by the other countries (Concerned Member State) involved.

Decentralized Procedure

This Decentralized procedure concerns when a product has not yet been authorized in any EU country and does not fall within centralized procedure, then companies can apply for the simultaneous authorization of the product in more than one EU country.

A dossier will be copied and circulated to all the EU countries in which marketing authorization is sought for the same product. The companies who submit the application are able to decide which country should be the 'Reference Member State' under this procedure.

The company (RMS) must prepare a preliminary report within 120 days and circulate it to every 'Concerned Member State'.

12.28   Pharmacology

Pharmacology is the branch of medicine concerned with the uses, effects, and modes of action of drugs.

Pharmacology is the study of drug and their interaction with the living organism.

The two main areas of pharmacology are :

- Pharmacodynamics

- Pharmacokinetics

Pharmacodynamics (PD) studies the effects of the drug on biological systems, and Pharmacokinetics (PK) studies the effects of biological systems on the drug.

In other words, PD can be defined as what drug does to body and PK can be defined as what the body does to drug.

Pharmacodynamics

Pharmacodynamics is the study of how a drug acts on a living organism, including the pharmacologic response and the duration and magnitude of response observed relative to the concentration of the drug at an active site in the organism.

Pharmacokinetics

Pharmacokinetics is the study of the processes (in a living organism) of absorption, distribution, metabolism, and excretion (ADME) of a drug.

- Absorption (A) - the process of a substance entering the blood circulation.

- Distribution (D) - the dispersion or dissemination of substances throughout the fluid and tissues of the body.

- Metabolism(M) - irreversible biotransformation

- Excretion (E) - the removal of the substances from the body

Absorption

Absorption of drug into the body system is required for showing its effect. Two main factors determines absorption:

- Route of administration
- Physiological factors which includes
    - Blood flow to the absorption site(high circulation-high absorption)
    - Total surface area (large area - more absorption)
    - Contact time (more contact time -more absorption)
    - Solubility (highly soluble -readily absorb in circulation), etc.

Distribution

When drug has entered and absorbed, it has to be distributed to the site of action or throughout the body. Elements of distribution:

- Distribution to the body fluid
- Distribution to the specific tissue/organ(e.g. iodine to Thyroid gland)
- Extent of plasma protein binding (e.g. Warfarin bound 97% to plasma protein)

Metabolism

Drug alteration in a living organism is known as biotransformation. Methods of biotransformation are:

- Non-synthetic Reactions (Phase I Reactions) - Oxidation, Reduction and Hydrolysis.
- Synthetic Reactions (Phase II Reactions) - Conjugation

Excretion

Drugs may be excreted in an active or inactive form. Various routes include Kidney, Lungs, Skin, Intestine, Saliva, etc.

Pharmacology is not to be confused with pharmacy. Pharmacy is a professional field in medicine concerned with preparation and distribution of medicine. Pharmacology is the study of the interaction and effects between chemicals and biological systems and vice versa.

Thirteen

ACTIVITY ASSIGNMENTS

- Find out difference between adverse reactions and side effects?

- Find out Regulatory Authority names for the following: USA, UK, France, Japan, Australia, Brazil, India, Europe, Canada

- Identify the reporter: "A nurse reported to the MAH that a pharmacist had reported that the patient experienced severe headache and rashes on face while on the medication".

- In the EU the EVCTM is used to facilitate the electronic reporting of Suspected Unexpected Serious Adverse Reactions (SUSARs). What does EVCTM stand for?

- Find out difference between High blood pressure and Hypertension?

- Write about ICH guidelines.

- What are different routes of drug administration?

- Find out some possible benefits and risks associated with taking part in a clinical trial?

- Find out two drugs used to treat hypertension and two drugs used to treat cardiac arrhythmias?

- Find out the difference between Clinical Practice and Clinical Research?

- Practice reporting adverse effects if any experienced after use of any medicinal product.

Fourteen

CAREERS IN DRUG SAFETY/PV

14.1   Learnings from the chapter

- *Relevant competencies/skills/knowledge required to make a good and progressive career in the field of pharmacovigilance/drug safety*

- *Selection process followed by companies to recruit professionals for pharmacovigilance/drug safety jobs*

- *HR Round of Interview: Personality traits which determine the overall employability chances of a candidate*

- *Various Job roles/positions in the field of pharmacovigilance/drug safety*

- *General Responsibiities - PV/drug safety job positions*

- *Subject related interview questions*

14.2   Introduction

Phamacovigilance/Drug Safety departments of companies specialized in this field recruit resources from various backgrounds (medical field, Pharma field, Biotechnology, Microbiology and other life science related fields). The pharmacovigilance professional are expected to have the relevant competencies (in terms of knowledge, skills and attributes) which are required to work efficiently in their respective drug safety job positions. This chapter focuses on the relevant competencies with respect to the drug safety jobs.

14.3 General Competencies for positions in Pharmacovigilance/drug safety jobs

Competencies	Description
Subject Knowledge	Ability to read and comprehend the clinical/scientific reports on pharmaceutical products.
	Good working knowledge of medical/clinical terminologies
	Good understanding of current FDA/ICH regulations pertaining to drug safety and pharmacovigilance
	Ability to understand the Pharmaceutical industry with regards to business perspective as well as the regulatory compliance requirements
	Understanding of the legal context such as data protection, copyright, patent etc
Analytical and Data related Skills	Ability to analyse and interpret the data pertaining to drug safety in relation to the benefit-risk assessment of the pharmaceutical product thereby providing the necessary insights which can be used to make the critical business decisions.
	Ability to present complex data in an understandable format
Communication/Comprehension	Excellent communication skills (both verbal and written)
	Ability to comprehend and communicate the information precisely and clearly.
Documentation/Reporting skills	Ability to clearly document in the written form for sharing the information with the manufacturer and with the regulatory authorities.
	Ability to write accurate and high quality reports.
	Ability of questioning and understanding in order to record the data accurately
Ethics	Ability to understand the sensitivity towards good vigilance practices modules and other pharmacovigilance guidelines
Value addition & Self Development	Ability to add value by identifying and working on the improvement areas as well as new areas - for development of self/team/department.
	Ability to Scale up in all competencies (knowledge, skills, attributes)
	Ability to keep oneself updated on latest developments on the regulatory requirements.
Other Competencies and Interpersonal Skills	Ability to plan, organize and prioritise the work on the basis of urgency of delivery of work and the compliance requirements
	Ability to work in a team environment
	Ability to work in remote organization and international cross-functional teams
	Ability to operate in target based assignments
	Problem solving skills
	Ability to manage multiple and varied tasks and prioritize workload with attention to detail
	Ability to source information
	Excellent Computer Skills - Microsoft Office (Word, Excel, PowerPoint, Outlook) and Internet skills

Levels of Competency

There are four levels of competencies. Basic, Intermediate, Advanced, Expert (starting from the lowest). Try to measure yourself as to what is your current level with respect to the each of these competencies mentioned in the above table. Once you make the right judgement about your current standing, you can make an attempt to move to the higher levels of competencies which will help you to get growth in your career.

14.4   Selection Process - Pharmacovigilance/Drug Safety roles

Most of the companies offering jobs in the field of drug safety/PV have a selection process in place which tests the calibre of the candidates with respect to the competencies required for the job position. Few common assessment areas are mentioned in the below table.

Aptitude Test Area	Purpose
Quantitative Aptitude Test	Tests the candidate's ability to deal with numbers quickly and accurately. It also tests the problem solving ability.
Verbal Reasoning Test	Tests the ability to think constructively, accurately and quickly.
Non Verbal (diagrammatic) Tests	Tests the logical reasoning ability and measures your ability to infer a set of rules from a flowchart or sequence of diagrams and then to apply those rules to new situation.
Situation/Scenario based Tests	Scenario based tests assess how you approach situations encountered in the workplace.
Interview – Technical Round	Tests your knowledge on the Subject of PV
Interview (HR Round)	Tests the candidate's interpersonal skills, behavioral aspects, self-confidence, and motivation necessary for the job.
Computer Skills Tests	Tests mainly the proficiency in using MS Office Tools and internet tools apart from checking the typing accuracy.
Written - Descriptive Tests	Tests the language ability, email writing etc

Aptitude Tests

The mantra to perform well in the aptitude test is very simple "PRACTICE". Hence, at present if you are not very good at numbers, ratios, calculation, non-verbal reasoning, logical reasoning etc, do not worry. Simply start practicing and keep practicing. The more you practice the easier it becomes. You need to believe strongly that **"IT IS ALL ABOUT PRACTICE AND NOTHING ELSE"**.

Subject Knowledge: This is the backbone for any professional. You need to understand the subject in the context of practical application and be always updated on the latest developments in the domain.

14.5   HR Round of Interview - Personality traits for employability

A candidate is considered to be employable if he/she has the potential to be a good employee. HR round tests the candidate on employability factor mainly with regards to the personality traits of the candidate. Few such areas are mentioned below:

Personality Trait	Description
Honesty, Integrity, Dependability	Honesty and integrity helps in creating trust which is important for any resource to operate in an organization.
Hard working/Takes Responsibilities	There is no substitute to hard work. Hardworking employees are asset to any organization.
Cultural Fit	Is the candidate going to like the working with the current set of employees in the company?
Positive and Full of Energy, Enthusiasm	Necessary to perform, generate new ideas etc. Stagnant employees with low energy levels make the organization unproductive.
Self-Motivated	Takes the responsibilities happily. Looks at the challenges as opportunities rather than a problem.
Adaptable	Willing to adjust to changes
Ethical	Follows rules, policies. Likes only right and lawful activities.
Team Player	Ability to work with many people
Action/Decision Oriented	Can take decision and initiate the actions
Result oriented	Works to achieve results
Thought Clarity	Clarity in understanding

14.6   Job Positions - Drug Safety Professionals

There are various roles in drug safety/pharmacovigilance departments of companies operating in this field. The designations vary from company to company

- Drug Safety Associate

- Safety Surveillance Associate

- PV Associate

- Drug Safety Officer/Manager

- Drug Safety Project Manager

- Quality Associate - Drug Safety

- Drug Safety Regulatory Compliance Manager

- Subject Matter Expert - Medical Reviewer

- Pharmacovigilance Officer

- Drug Safety and Medical Affairs Executive

- Drug Safety Analyst

14.7   General Responsibiities - Pharmacovigilance/Drug Safety

What is the role of a drug safety/pharmacovigilance professional?

The generalized role encompasses the following. The role however may vary from company to company.

- Receiving, processing and reporting of adverse event reports.

- To obtain more details, a follow up with the reporters of adverse events is needed.

- Providing the required information on drug safety to the concerned parties.

- Providing support to the internal cross-functional teams in terms of drug safety expertise.

- Ensuring that the day to day pharmacovigilance processes are being followed correctly.

- Attending the safety related meetings.

- Looking in to the business angle of drug safety.

- Ensuring that Pharmacovigilance Quality compliance is met across the organisation

- Responsible for designing, implementing and maintaining the drug safety management programs. Establishing safety guidelines as well as ensuring proper safety databases and the quality of data input into those databases.

Note: The roles mentioned above is a generalized list and does not intend to cover the individual job positions mentioned in the section: Job Positions - Drug Safety Professionals.

14.8   General subject related questions helpful for interview preparation

- What is Pharmacovigilance?

- Define these terms: ADR, SAE, SUSAR, AE, IBD, PSUR, DSUR, Signal, DLP, DIBD, Off-label use, SmPC, ICSR.

- What are the different Phases of clinical trials?

- What is the minimum criteria for reporting?

- What is Unexpected adverse reaction and expected adverse reaction?

- What is MedDRA, it's current version, when it is updated? SOC, HLGT, HLT, PT, LLT'
- List the Countries and their regulatory authorities.
- What is Dechallenge and Rechallenge (Positive and Negative)?
- What is the Criteria for Expedited Reporting?
- What are the timelines of SAE reporting?
- What are the Reporting Forms used for different countries like Medwatch/yellow cards/CIOMS?
- What is meant by Day Zero?
- What is the difference between a health care professional and an non-healthcare professional?
- What is the difference between pre-marketing and post marketing studies?
- What is meant by post marketing surveillance?
- What is the difference between adverse event and adverse drug reaction?
- What are the SAE criteria?
- What are the various outcomes of SAE (worst to favourable outcome)?
- What is E2B reporting?
- List few types of post marketing studies.
- List few algorithm names.
- Mention the names of documents used to assess expectedness.

For any further assistance log on to the website pv.crinov.com or write at amrita@crinov.com

Glossary

Active Ingredient - the chemically active part of a chemical compound.

Adverse Drug Reaction (ADR) - is an unintended reaction occurring with a drug where a positive (direct) causal relationship between the event and the drug is thought, or has been proven, to exist.

Adverse event (AE) -any untoward medical occurrence in a patient or clinical investigation subject, administered a pharmaceutical product and which does not necessarily have to have a causal relationship with this treatment.

Allopath - non-traditional, western scientific therapy, usually using synthesised ingredients, but may also contain a purified active ingredient extracted from a plant or other natural source, usually in opposition to the disease.

Analogy - a comparison between one thing and another, typically for the purpose of explanation or clarification.

Animal model - is a living, non-human animal used during the research and investigation of human disease, for the purpose of better understanding the disease process without the added risk of harming an actual human.

Benefit-risk profile - description or analysis of whether the therapeutic benefits of using apharmaceutical product outweigh the risks involved. This balance can be different for certain groups of patients or for those with particular coexisting conditions/diseases.

Benefits - are commonly expressed as the proven therapeutic good of a product but should also include the patient's subjective assessment of its effects.

Bioequivalence - two pharmaceutical products are bioequivalent if they are pharmaceutically equivalent and their bioavailabilities (rate and extent of availability), after administration in the same molar dose, are similar to such a degree that their effects can be expected to be essentially the same.

Carcinogenicity - ability of a carcinogen (any substance or agent that tends to produce a cancer) to produce invasive cancer cells from normal cells.

Causal relationship - is said to exist when a drug is thought to have caused or contributed to the occurrence of an adverse drug reaction.

Clinical trial (or study) - refers to an organized program to determine the safety and/or efficacy of a drug (or drugs) in patients. The design of a clinical trial will depend on the drug and the phase of its development.

Cohort Event Monitoring (CEM) - is a prospective, observational study of events that occur during the use of medicines, for intensified follow-up of selected medicinal products phase. Patients are monitored from the time they begin treatment, and for a defined period of time.

Concomitant medication - a medicine taken concurrently with another medicine. This includes not only prescribed medicines, but also homeopathic treatments, herbal treatments, vitamins, and other non prescription medications.

Contractual agreement - an agreement between two or more parties, especially one that is written and enforceable by law.

CRO (Contract Research Organization) - a person or an organization (commercial, academic or other) contracted by the sponsor to perform one or more of a sponsor's study-related duties and functions.

Determinant - any factor that brings about change in a health condition, or other defined characteristic.

Dizziness - a term used to describe everything from feeling faint or lightheaded to feeling weak or unsteady.

Dose - the amount of medicine taken, or radiation given, at one time.

Dose-dependent - refers to the effects of treatment with a drug. If the effects change when the dose of the drug is changed, the effects are said to be dose-dependent.

Drug Interaction - is a situation in which a substance (usually another drug) affects the activity of a drug when both are administered together.

Drug Safety and Monitoring Board (DSMB) - an independent committee, composed of community representatives and clinical research experts, that reviews data while a clinical trial is in progress to ensure that participants are not exposed to undue risk. A DSMB may recommend that a trial be stopped if there are safety concerns or if the trial objectives have been achieved.

Drug utilization evaluation studies - studies which assess the appropriateness of drug use. They are designed to detect and quantify the frequency of drug use problems.

Effectiveness - is the extent to which a drug works under real world circumstances, i.e., clinical practice.

Efficacy - is the extent to which a drug works under ideal circumstances, i.e., in clinical trials.

Endogenous - proceeding from within; derived internally.

Epidemiology - is the branch of medical science that deals with the study of incidence, distribution and control of a disease in a population.

Equilibrium of body - is the ability of the body or a cell to seek and maintain a condition of equilibrium or stability within its internal environment when dealing with external changes.

Ethics Committee - an independent group of both medical and non-medical professionals who are responsible for verifying the integrity of a study and ensuring the safety, integrity, and human rights of the study participants.

Expedited report/reporting - is safety reports that require reporting within short timeframes to regulatory authorities (such as the FDA in the U.S. or the EMA in Europe). The specific requirements may vary by regulatory agency, but factors typically include the seriousness of the specific adverse event, whether it would be expected to occur and whether it might be related to an investigational medicine.

Gene chip technology - is development of cDNA microarrays from a large number of genes. Used to monitor and measure changes in gene expression for each gene represented on the chip.

Genome - the complete set of genes or genetic material present in a cell or organism.

Genomics - study of genomes (the complete set of genes or genetic material present in a cell or organism).

Harm - is the nature and extent of the actual damage that could be or has been caused.

Hazards - a danger or risk.

HCP (Healthcare professional) - is a medically-qualified person such as a physician, dentist, pharmacist, nurse, coroner, or as otherwise specified by local regulations.

Herbal medicine - includes herbs, herbal materials, herbal preparations and finished herbal products.

Homeopathy - is a therapeutic system which works on the principle that 'like treats like'. An illness is treated with a medicine which could produce similar symptoms in a healthy person. The active ingredients are given in highly diluted form to avoid toxicity. Homeopathic remedies are virtually 100% safe.

Implied causality - refers to spontaneously reported AE cases where the causality is always presumed to be positive unless the reporter states otherwise.

In vitro - in the laboratory (outside the body), opposite of in vivo (in the body).

In vivo - in the body, opposite of in vitro (outside the body or in the laboratory).

Incidence - number of new cases of an outcome which develop over a defined time period in a defined population at risk.

Indication - a symptom that suggests certain medical treatment is necessary.

Individual Case Safety Report (ICSR) - a report that contains information describing a suspected adverse drug reaction related to the administration of one or more medicinal product ucts to an individual patient.

Inpatient - a patient who lives in hospital while under treatment.

Investigational new drug (IND) - a new drug, antibiotic drug or biological drug, that is used in a clinical investigation. It also includes a biological product used in vitro for diagnostic purposes.

Investigator - a medical professional, usually a physician but may also be a nurse, pharmacist or other health care professional, under whose direction an investigational drug is administered or dispensed.

Lead - a lead compound (i.e. a "leading" compound, not lead metal) in drug discovery is a chemical compound that has pharmacological or biological activity likely to be therapeutically useful, but may still have suboptimal structure that requires modification to fit better to the target.

Life-threatening - refers to an adverse event that places a patient at the immediate risk of death.

Ligand - a molecule that binds to another (usually larger) molecule.

MAH (Marketing Authorization holder) -is usually an organization to whom permission has been granted for marketing the medicinal product (s) for specified indication. It has an appropriate system of pharmacovigilance in place in order to assure responsibility and liability for its products on the market and to ensure that appropriate action can be taken, when necessary.

Manufacturer - a person or company that makes products/goods for sale.

Marketing authorization - an official document issued by the competent drug regulatory authority for the purpose of marketing or free distribution of a product after evaluation for safety, efficacy and quality.

Medical History - a narrative or record of past events and circumstances that are or may be relevant to a patient's current state of health. Informally, an account of past diseases, injuries, treatments, and other strictly medical facts.

MedWatch - a system maintained by the U.S. Food & Drug Administration (FDA) for the voluntary reporting of adverse events, potential and actual medical product errors, and product quality problems associated with the use of FDA-regulated medicines, biologics, devices, and dietary supplements.

Member countries - countries which comply with the criteria for, and have joined the WHO Programme for International Drug Monitoring.

Microarray - are simply ordered sets of DNA molecules of known sequence provide pharmaceutical firms with a means to identify drug targets.

Monitoring - is the performance and analysis of routine measurements aimed at detecting changes in the environment or health status of populations.

Morbidity - refers to the disease state of an individual, or the incidence of illness in a population.

Mortality - refers to the state of being mortal, or the incidence of death (number of deaths) in a population.

Mutagenicity - is the property of a physical, biological or chemical agent (a mutagen) to induce genetic mutation. A mutagen may act directly on the DNA, causing direct damage to the DNA, and most often result in replication error.

National pharmacovigilance centers - are organizations recognized by governments to represent their country in the WHO Programme (usually the drug regulatory agency). A single, governmentally recognized centre (or integrated system) within a country with the clinical and scientific expertise to collect, collate, analyze and give advice on all information related to drug safety.

Non-HCP (Non-healthcare professional) - is defined as a person who is not a healthcare professional such as a patient, lawyer, friend, or relative of a patient.

Nucleic Acid - a complex organic substance present in living cells, especially DNA or RNA, whose molecules consist of many nucleotides linked in a long chain.

Opoids - is any chemical that resembles morphine or other opiates in its pharmacological effects

OTC (Over The Counter) medicine - medicinal product available to the public without prescription.

Outpatient - a patient who visits a health care facility for diagnosis or treatment without spending the night,. sometimes called a day patient.

Pharmacoeconomics - refers to the scientific discipline that compares the value of one pharmaceutical drug or drug therapy to another. It is a sub-discipline of health economics.

Pharmacological effects - may be defined as the physiological and/or biochemical changes in the body produced by a drug in therapeutic concentration. No drug has a single pharmacological effect. A drug usually produces several pharmacological effects. Pharmacological effects may be classified as desired and undesired effects even when used in usual dose. For example, rifampicin is used for the treatment of tuberculosis. The desired effect of this drug is to kill the causative microorganism Mycobacterium tuberculosis so that the patient will be cured from tuberculosis. But the therapeutic concentration of rifampicin also causes some undesirable effects that are not avoidable.Undesired effects may be harmless, harmful, or beneficial. For example, one undesired effect of rifampicin is that it alters the color of urine, feces, sweats, and tears to red-orange and this effect is harmless.

Plausibility - the quality or state of being plausible (seeming likely to be true, or able to be believed) **Post-marketing** - the stage when a drug is generally available on the market.

Pre-marketing - the stage before a drug is available for prescription or sale to the public.

Prescription Event Monitoring (PEM) - system created to monitor adverse drug events in a population. Prescribers are requested to report all events, regardless of whether they are suspected adverse events, for identified patients receiving a specified drug.

Prescription Only Medicine (POM) - medicinal product available to the public only on prescription.

Prevalence - number of existing cases of an outcome in a defined population at a given point in time.

Prophylaxis - prevention or protection.

Proteome - entire set of proteins expressed by a genome, cell, tissue or organism at a certain time.

Proteomics - the study of proteomes (entire set of proteins expressed by a genome, cell, tissue or organism at a certain time) and their functions.

Rational drug use - an ideal of therapeutic practice in which drugs are prescribed and used in exact accordance with the best understanding of their appropriateness for the indication and the particular patient, and of their benefit, harm effectiveness and risk.

Record linkage - method of assembling information contained in two or more records, e.g in different sets of medical charts, and in vital records such as birth and death certificates. This makes it possible to relate significant health events that are remote from one another in time and place.

Registry - is a system of ongoing registration in which data are collected concerning all cases of a particular disease or other health-relevant condition in a defined population such that the case can be related to a population base. Examples include cancer registries, birth defect registries and death registries.

Regulatory Authority - also known as regulatory agency/ regulatory body or regulator, i a public authority or government agency responsible for exercising autonomous authority ove some area of human activity in a regulatory or supervisory capacity.

Risk - the probability that an event will occur.

Risk factors - is any attribute, characteristic or exposure of an individual that increases the likelihood of developing a disease or injury.

Safety - relative freedom from harm

Sample Size - a subset of a larger population, selected for investigation to draw conclusions o make estimates about the larger population.

Serendipity - Serendipity is when someone accidently finds something good.(e.g. Penicillin)

Side effect - Any unintended effect of a pharmaceutical product occurring at normal dosag which is related to the pharmacological properties of the drug.

Sponser - individual, company, institution or organization taking responsibility for initia tion, management and financing of study.

Subject - a patient or healthy individual participating in a research study voluntarily.

Summary of Product Characteristics (SPC) - is a regulatory document attached to the marketing authorization which forms the basis of the product information made available to prescribers and patients.

Surveillance - is ongoing scrutiny, generally using methods distinguished by their practicability, uniformity, and rapidity, rather than by complete accuracy. Its main purpose is to detect changes in trends or distribution in order to initiate investigative or control measures.

Survey - to query (someone) in order to collect data for the analysis of some aspect of a group or area.

Syndrome - a group of symptoms which consistently occur together, or a condition characterized by a set of associated symptoms.

Target - is the naturally existing cellular or molecular structure involved in the pathology (the science of the causes and effects of diseases) of interest that the drug-in-development is meant to act on.

Temporal relationship - is said to exist when an adverse event occurs when a patient is taking a given drug. Although a temporal relationship is absolutely necessary in order to establish a causal relationship between the drug and the AE, a temporal relationship does not necessarily in and of itself prove that the event was caused by the drug.

Teratogenicity - is the ability to cause developmental anomalies in a fetus. Things that can cause developmental abnormalities are known as teratogens, and they include things like viruses, chemicals, and radiation. Their study is known as teratology.

Toxicity - having the capability to cause death or injury. May pertain to an adverse event produced by a medicine that is detrimental to the subject's health. The level of toxicity associated with a medicine may vary with the condition for which the medicine is used, as well as the dosage used.

Toxicology - the study of the potential for a substance (e.g., a medicine) to have toxic (i.e., harmful) effects on the body.

Treatment - an act or manner of treating (to deal with a disease,patient,etc.) in order to relieve or cure.

Triage - refers to the process of placing a potential adverse event report into one of three categories: 1) non-serious case; 2) serious case; or 3) no case (minimum criteria for an AE case are not fulfilled).

Verbatim - in exactly the same words as were used originally.

Verification - is a process to ensure that the data contained in final report matches with original observations.

Vulnerable population - are defined as those at greater risk for poor health status and health care access.

WHO Drug Dictionary (WHO DD) - the WHO Drug Dictionary is an international classification of drugs providing proprietary and on-proprietary names of medicinal products used in different countries, together with all active ingredients.

WHO-ART - terminology for coding clinical information in relation to drug therapy. WHO ART is maintained by UMC.

Printed in Great Britain
by Amazon